The Definitive Diabetic Collection to Tea and Infusion for Beginners

Tasty and Refreshing Drinks to Boost Your Metabolism and Enjoy Relaxing Moments

D1794896

Braylee Hester

1

contained within this document, including, but not limited to, — errors, omissions, or inaccuracies.

Table of contents

Kale Smoothie

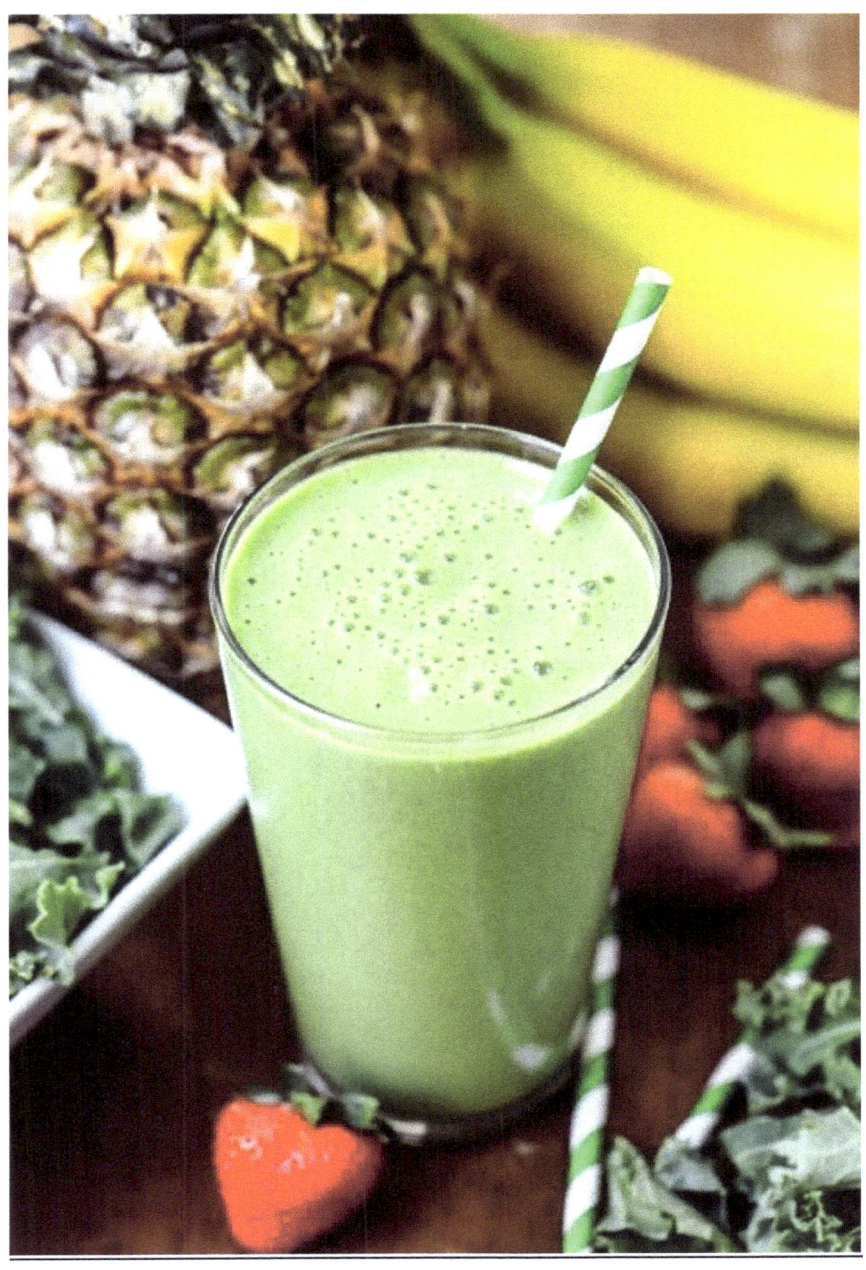

Preparation Time : 10 minutes
Cooking Time : 0 minutes

Servings : 2

Ingredients :

- 3 stalks fresh kale, trimmed and chopped
- 1-2 celery stalks, chopped
- ½ avocado, peeled, pitted, and chopped
- ½-inch piece ginger root, chopped
- ½-inch piece turmeric root, chopped
- 2 cups coconut milk

Directions :

1. Place all the ingredients in a high-speed blender and pulse until creamy.
2. Pour the smoothie into two glasses and serve immediately.

Nutrition : Calories 248; Total Fat 21.8 g; Saturated Fat 12 g; Cholesterol 0 mg; Sodium 59 mg; Total Carbs 11.3 g; Fiber 4.2 g; Sugar 0.5 g, Protein 3.5 g

Green Tofu Smoothie

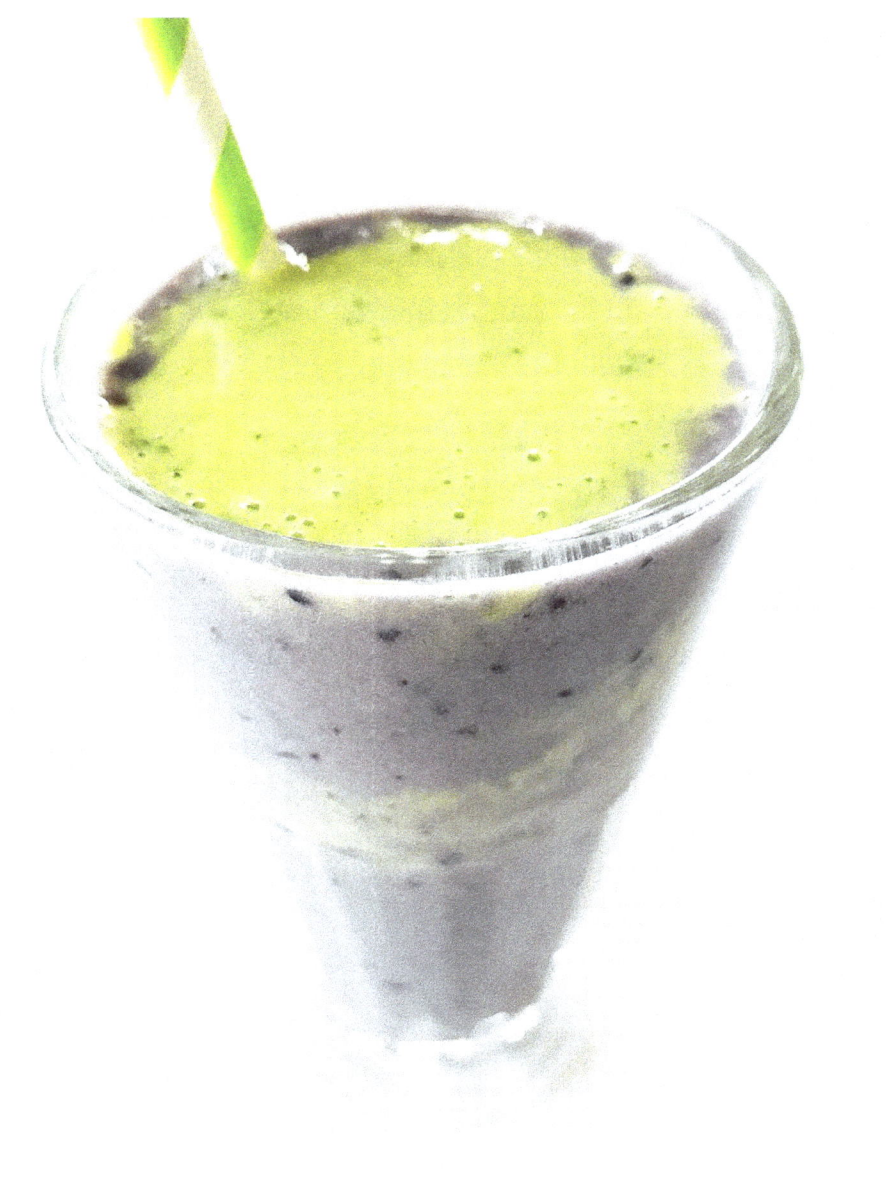

Preparation   Time   :   10   minutes
 Cooking Time : 0 minutes

Servings : 2

Ingredients :

- 1½ cups cucumber, peeled and chopped roughly
- 3 cups fresh baby spinach
- 2 cups frozen broccoli
- ½ cup silken tofu, drained and pressed
- 1 tablespoon fresh lime juice
- 4-5 drops liquid stevia
- 1 cup unsweetened almond milk
- ½ cup ice, crushed

Directions :

1. Place all the ingredients in a high-speed blender and pulse until creamy.
2. Pour the smoothie into two glasses and serve immediately.

Nutrition : Calories 118; Total Fat 15 g; Saturated Fat 0.8 g; Cholesterol 0 mg; Sodium 165 mg; Total Carbs 12.6 g; Fiber 4.8 g; Sugar 3.4 g; Protein 10 g

Grape & Swiss Chard Smoothie

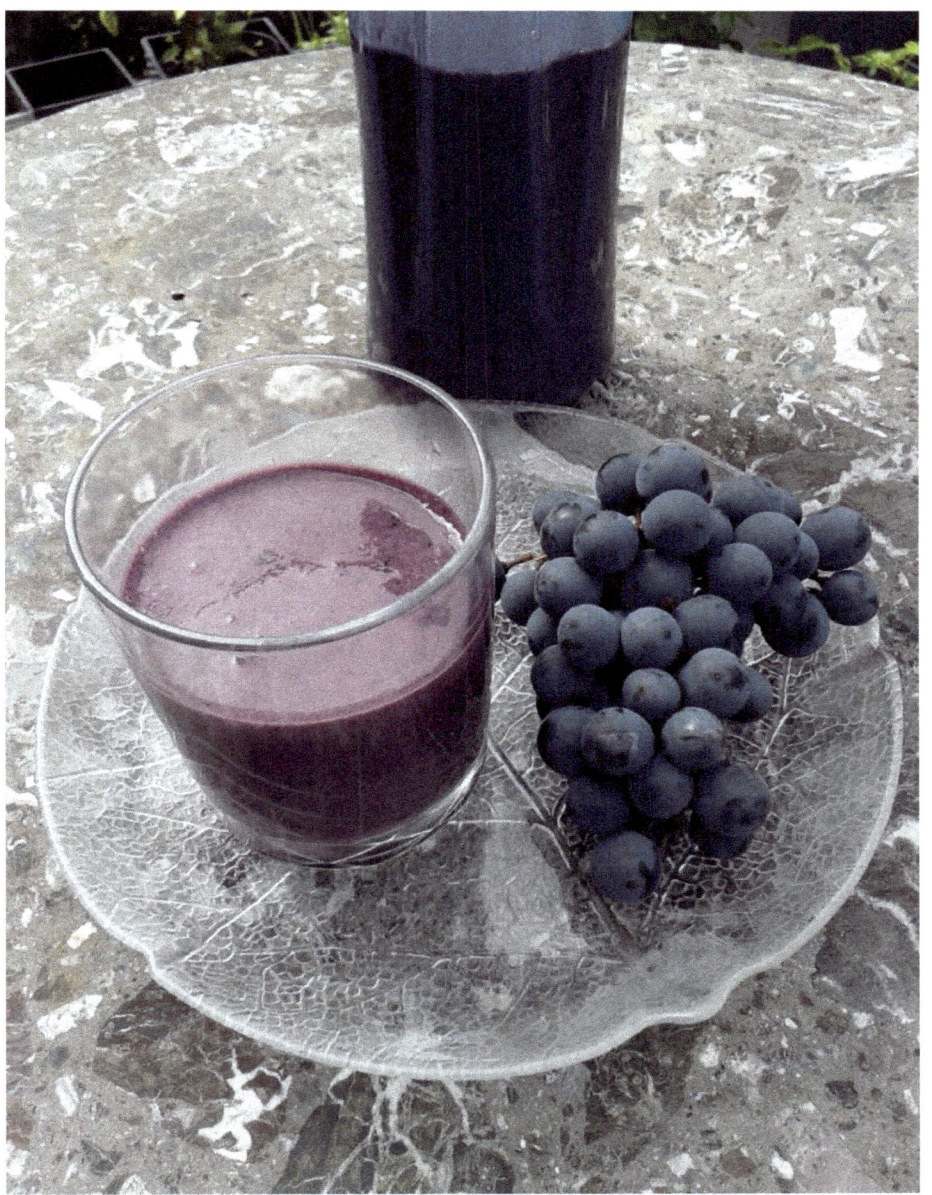

Preparation Time : 10 minutes
Cooking Time : 0 minutes

Servings : 2

Ingredients :

- 2 cups seedless green grapes
- 2 cups fresh Swiss chard, trimmed and chopped
- 2 tablespoons maple syrup
- 1 teaspoon fresh lemon juice
- 1½ cups water
- 4 ice cubes

Directions :

1. Place all the ingredients in a high-speed blender and pulse until creamy.
2. Pour the smoothie into two glasses and serve immediately.

Nutrition : Calories 176; Total Fat 0.2 g; Saturated Fat 0 g; Cholesterol 0 mg; Sodium 83 mg; Total Carbs 44.9 g; Fiber 1.7 g; Sugar 37.9 g; Protein 0.7 g

Matcha Smoothie

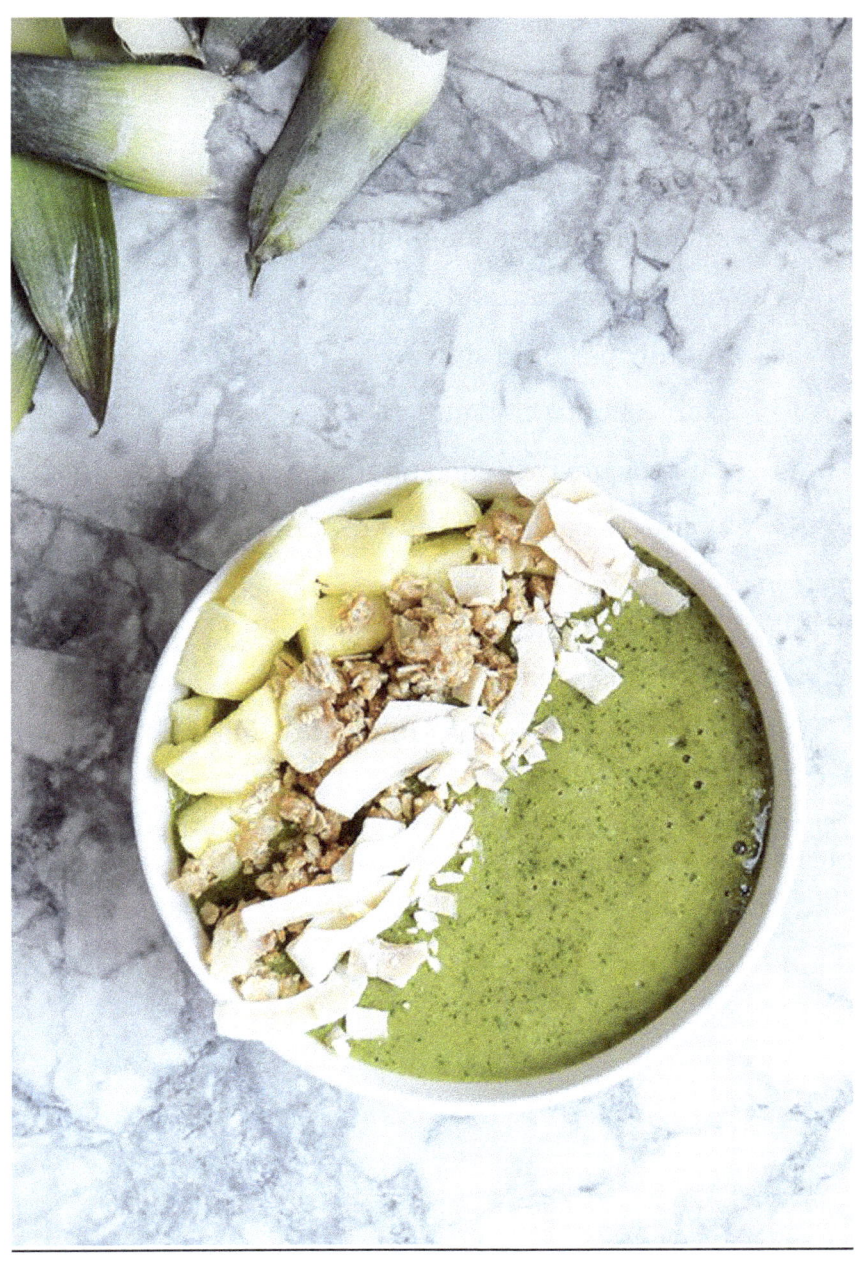

Preparation Time : 10 minutes

Cooking   Time   :   0   minutes
Servings : 2

Ingredients :

- 2 tablespoons chia seeds
- 2 teaspoons matcha green tea powder
- ½ teaspoon fresh lemon juice
- ½ teaspoon xanthan gum
- 8-10 drops liquid stevia
- 4 tablespoons coconut cream
- 1½ cups unsweetened almond milk
- ¼ cup ice cubes

Directions :

1. Place all the ingredients in a high-speed blender and pulse until creamy.

2. Pour the smoothie into two glasses and serve immediately.

Nutrition : Calories 132; Total Fat 12.3 g; Saturated Fat 6.8 g; Cholesterol 0 mg; Sodium 15 mg; Total Carbs 7 g; Fiber 4.8 g; Sugar 1 g; Protein 3 g

Banana Smoothie

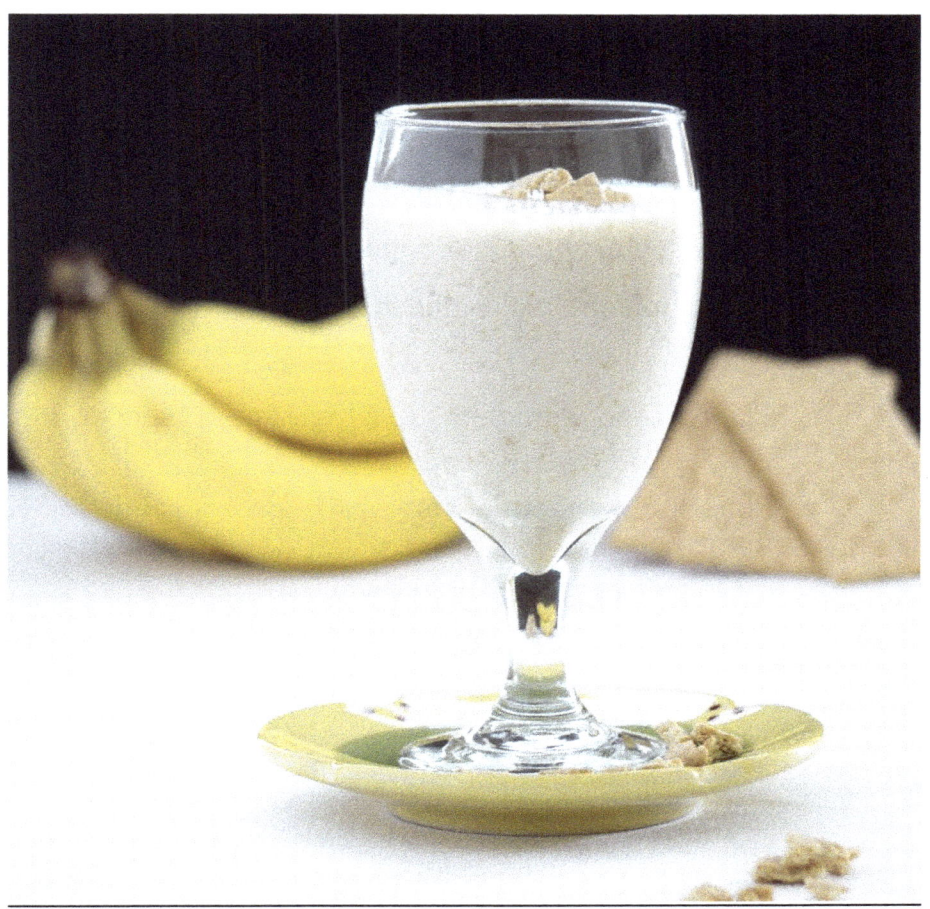

Preparation Time : 10 minutes

Cooking   Time   :   0   minutes
Servings : 2

Ingredients :

- 2 cups chilled unsweetened almond milk
- 1 large frozen banana, peeled and sliced
- 1 tablespoon almonds, chopped
- 1 teaspoon organic vanilla extract

Directions :

1. Place all the ingredients in a high-speed blender and pulse until creamy.
2. Pour the smoothie into two glasses and serve immediately.

Nutrition : Calories 124; Total Fat 5.2 g; Saturated Fat 0.5 g; Cholesterol 0 mg; Sodium 181 mg; Total Carbs 18.4 g; Fiber 3.1 g; Sugar 8.7 g; Protein 2.4 g

Strawberry Smoothie

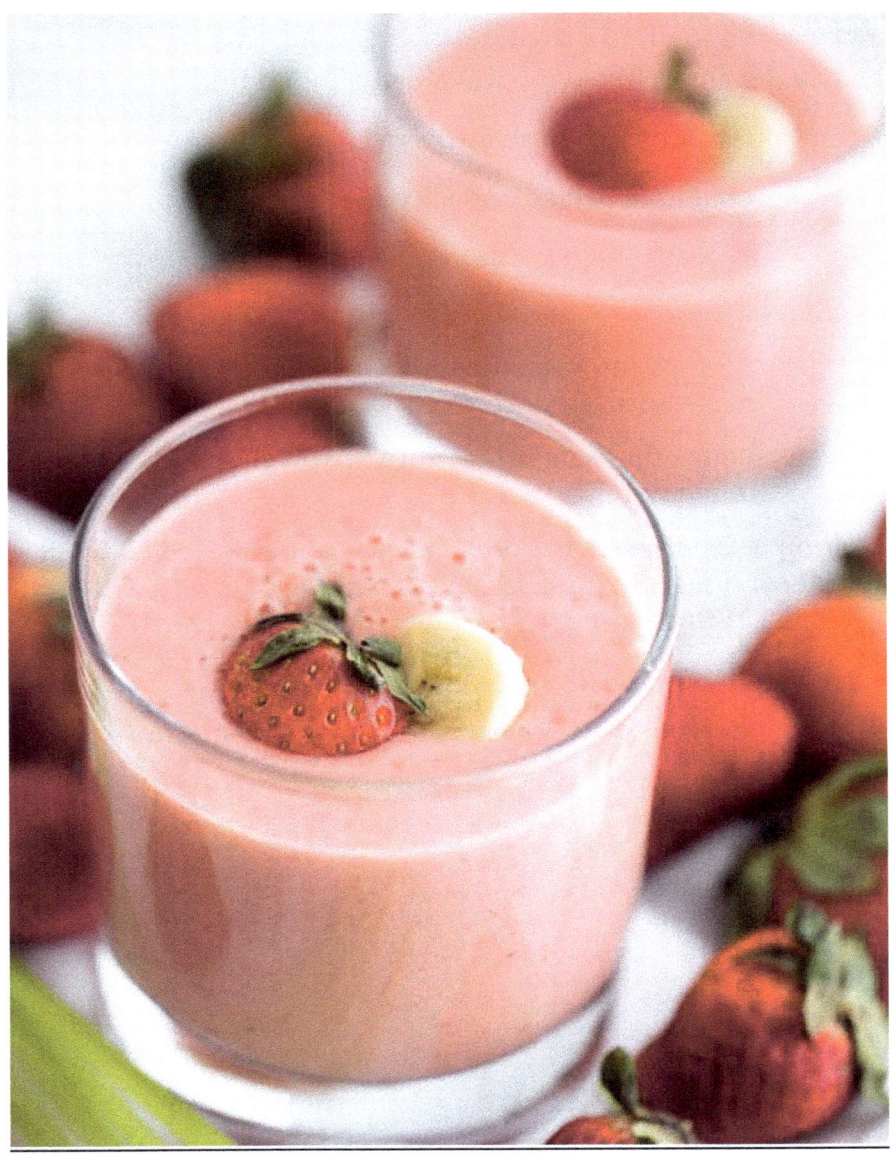

Preparation Time : 10 minutes

Cooking Time : 0 minutes

Servings : 2

Ingredients :

- 2 cups chilled unsweetened almond milk

- 1½ cups frozen strawberries

- 1 banana, peeled and sliced

- ¼ teaspoon organic vanilla extract

Directions :

1. Add all the ingredients in a high-speed blender and pulse until smooth.

2. Pour the smoothie into two glasses and serve immediately.

Nutrition : Calories 131; Total Fat 3.7 g; Saturated Fat 0.4 g; Cholesterol 0 mg; Sodium 181 mg; Total Carbs 25.3 g; Fiber 4.8 g; Sugar 14 g; Protein 1.6 g

Raspberry & Tofu Smoothie

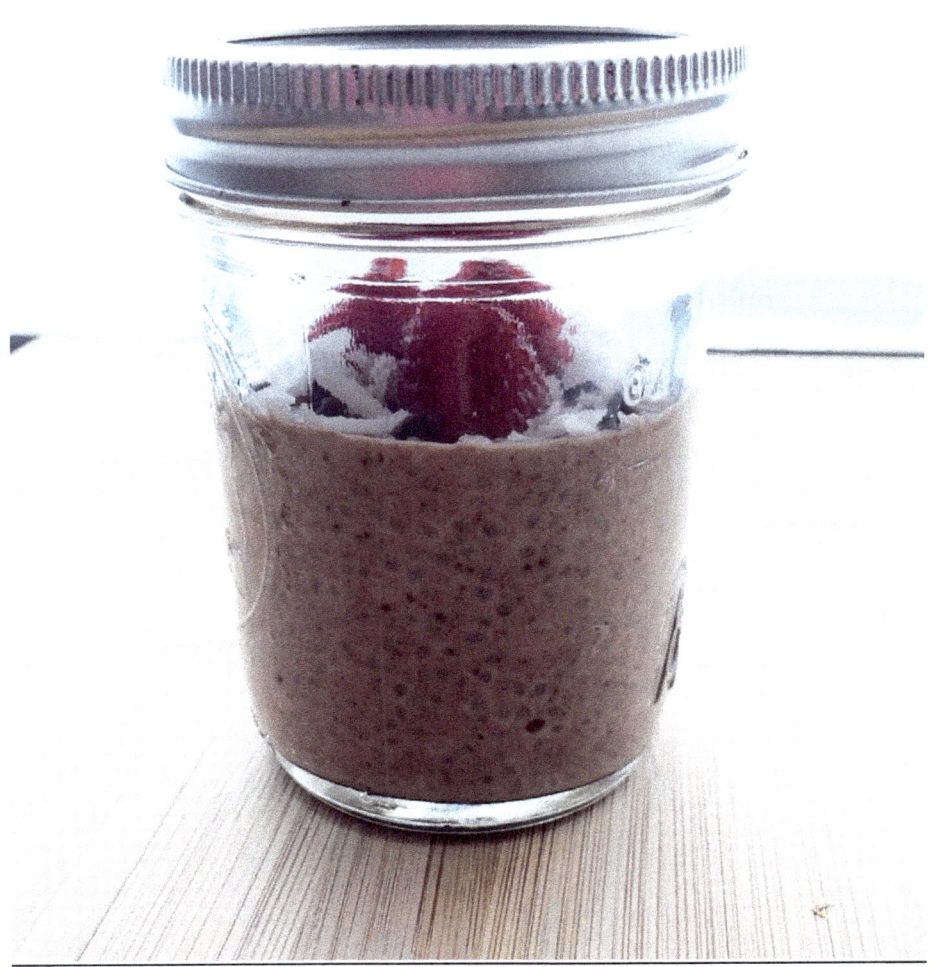

Preparation Time : 15 minutes

Cooking Time : 0 minutes

Servings : 2

Ingredients :

- 1½ cups fresh raspberries
- 6 ounces firm silken tofu, drained
- 1/8 teaspoon coconut extract
- 1 teaspoon powdered stevia
- 1½ cups unsweetened almond milk
- ¼ cup ice cubes, crushed

Directions :

1. Add all the ingredients in a high-speed blender and pulse until smooth.
2. Pour the smoothie into two glasses and serve immediately.

Nutrition : Calories 131; Total Fat 5.5 g; Saturated Fat 0.6 g; Cholesterol 0 mg; Sodium 167 mg; Total Carbs 14.6 g; Fiber 6.8 g; Sugar 5.2 g, Protein 7.7 g

Mango Smoothie

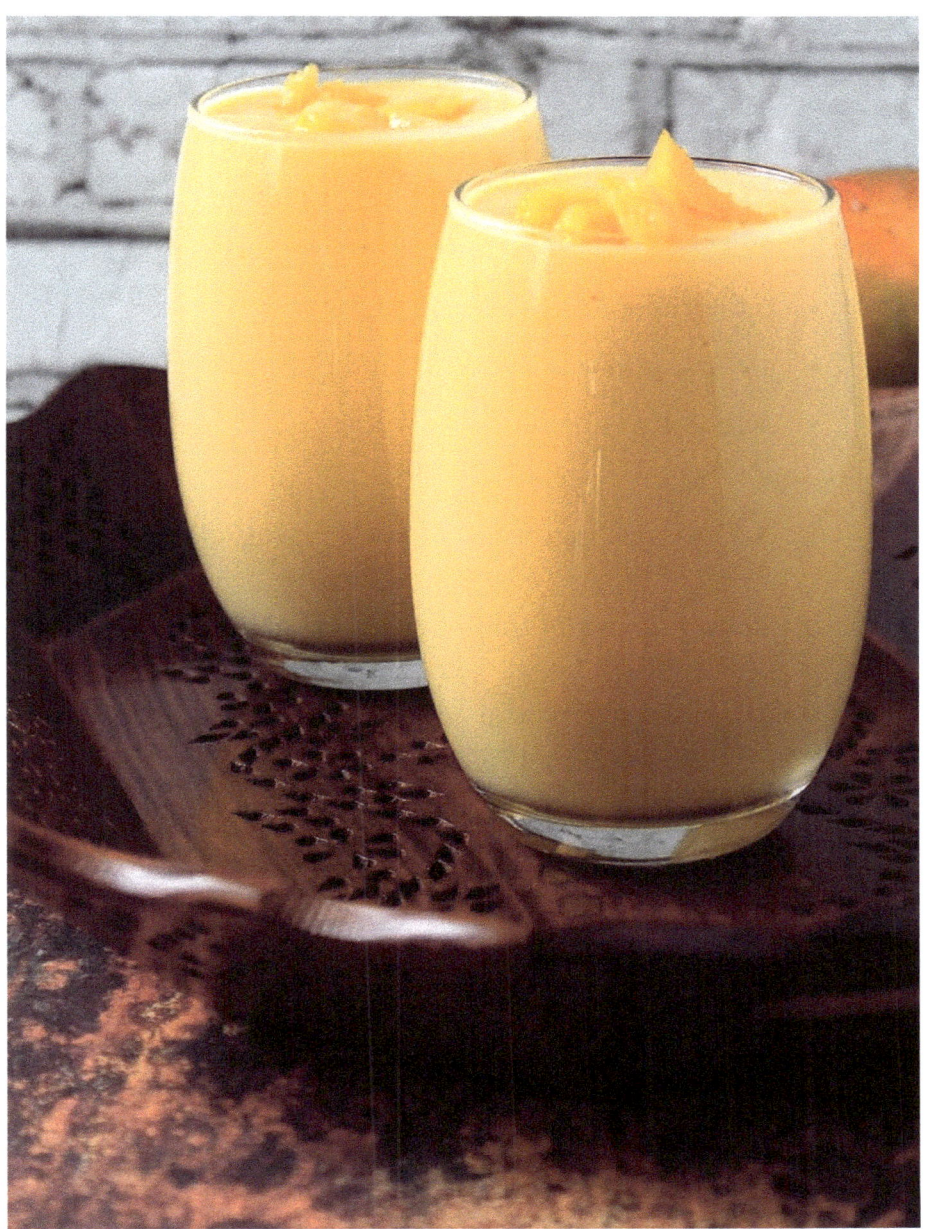

Preparation Time : 10 minutes

Cooking   Time   :   0   minutes
 Servings : 2

Ingredients :

- 2 cups frozen mango, peeled, pitted and chopped

- ¼ cup almond butter

- Pinch of ground turmeric

- 2 tablespoons fresh lemon juice

- 1¼ cups unsweetened almond milk

- ¼ cup ice cubes

Directions :

1. Add all the ingredients in a high-speed blender and pulse until smooth.

2. Pour the smoothie into two glasses and serve immediately.

Nutrition : Calories 140; Total Fat 4.1 g; Saturated Fat 0.6 g; Cholesterol 0 mg; Sodium 118 mg; Total Carbs 26.8 g; Fiber 3.6 g; Sugar 23 g; Protein 2.5 g

Pineapple Smoothie

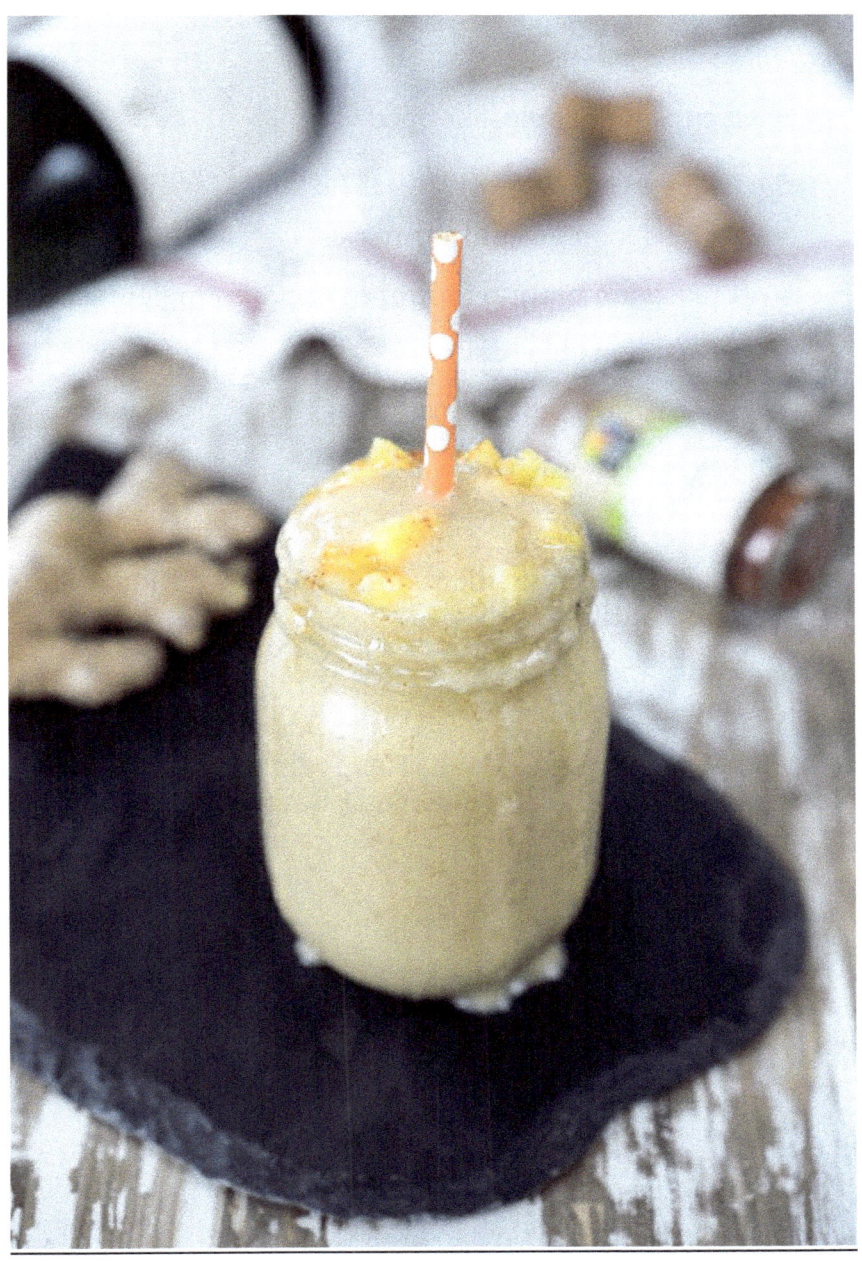

Preparation Time : 10 minutes

Cooking   Time   :   0   minutes
 Servings : 2

Ingredients :

- 2 cups pineapple, chopped
- ½ teaspoon fresh ginger, peeled and chopped
- ½ teaspoon ground turmeric
- 1 teaspoon natural immune support supplement *
- 1 teaspoon chia seeds
- 1½ cups cold green tea
- ½ cup ice, crushed

Directions :

1. Add all the ingredients in a high-speed blender and pulse until smooth.

2. Pour the smoothie into two glasses and serve immediately.

Nutrition : Calories 152; Total Fat 1 g; Saturated Fat 0 g; Cholesterol 0 mg; Sodium 9 mg; Total Carbs 30 g; Fiber 3.5 g; Sugar 29.8 g; Protein 1.5 g

Kale & Pineapple Smoothie

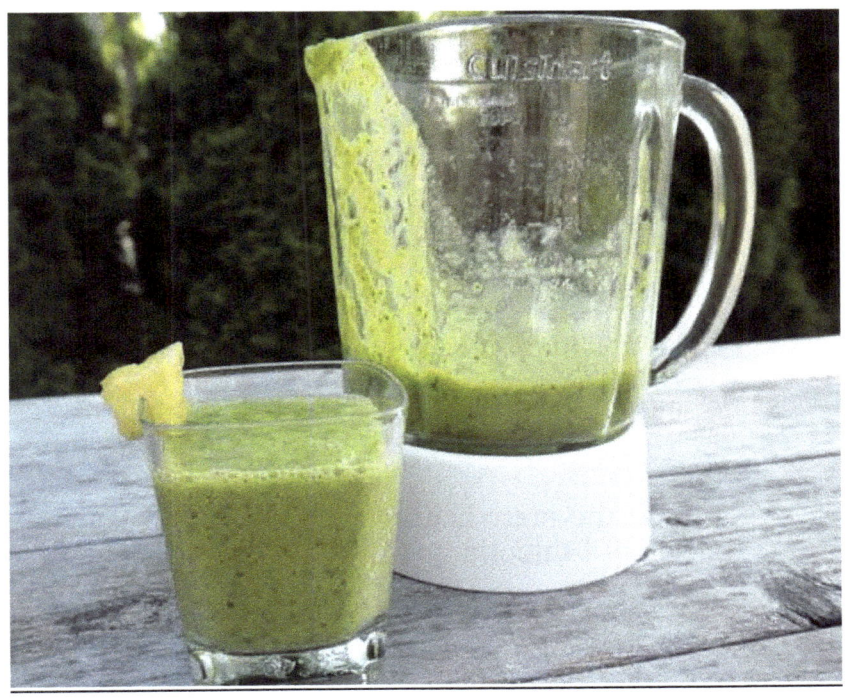

Preparation Time : 15 minutes

Cooking   Time   :   0   minutes
Servings : 2

Ingredients :

- 1½ cups fresh kale, trimmed and chopped
- 1 frozen banana, peeled and chopped
- ½ cup fresh pineapple chunks
- 1 cup unsweetened coconut milk
- ½ cup fresh orange juice
- ½ cup ice

Directions :

1. Add all the ingredients in a high-speed blender and pulse until smooth.

2. Pour the smoothie into two glasses and serve immediately.

Nutrition : Calories 148; Total Fat 2.4 g; Saturated Fat 2.1 g; Cholesterol 0 mg; Sodium 23 mg; Total Carbs 31.6 g; Fiber 3.5 g; Sugar 16.5 g; Protein 2.8 g

Green Veggies Smoothie

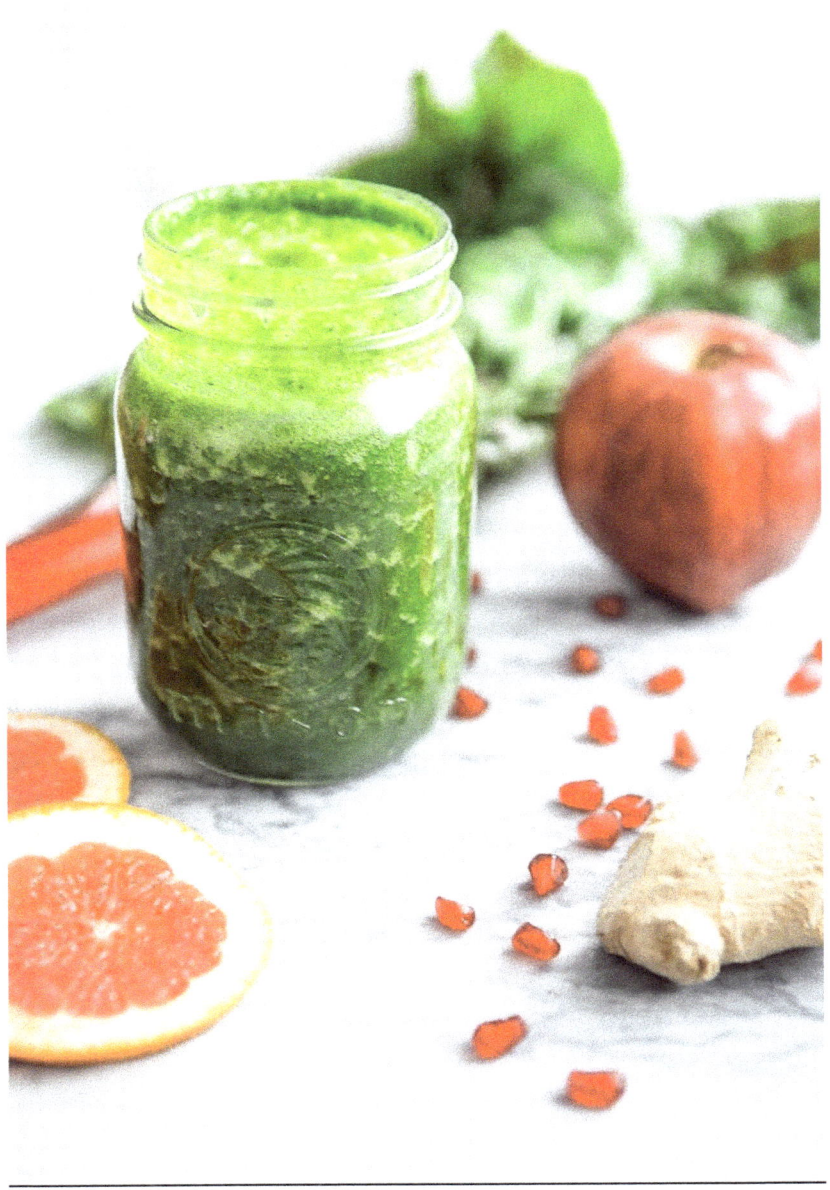

Preparation Time : 15 minutes

Cooking Time : 0 minutes
Servings : 2

Ingredients :

- 1 medium avocado, peeled, pitted, and chopped
- 1 large cucumber, peeled and chopped
- 2 fresh tomatoes, chopped
- 1 small green bell pepper, seeded and chopped
- 1 cup fresh spinach, torn
- 2 tablespoons fresh lime juice
- 2 tablespoons homemade vegetable broth
- 1 cup alkaline water

Directions :

1. Add all the ingredients in a high-speed blender and pulse until smooth.
2. Pour the smoothie into glasses and serve immediately.

Nutrition : Calories 275; Total Fat 20.3 g; Saturated Fat 4.2 g; Cholesterol 0 mg; Sodium 76 mg; Total Carbs 24.1 g; Fiber 10.1 g; Sugar 9.3 g; Protein 5.3 g

Avocado & Spinach Smoothie

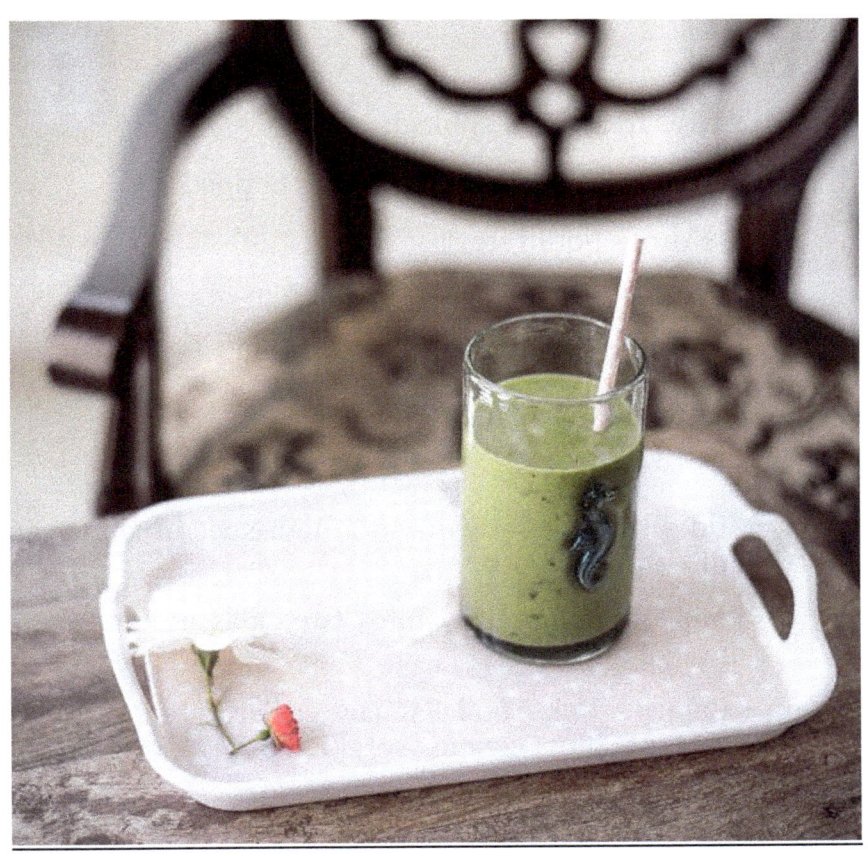

Preparation Time : 10 minutes

Cooking   Time   :   0   minutes
Servings : 2

Ingredients :

- 2 cups fresh baby spinach
- ½ avocado, peeled, pitted, and chopped
- 4-6 drops liquid stevia
- ½ teaspoon ground cinnamon
- 1 tablespoon hemp seeds
- 2 cups chilled alkaline water

Directions :

1. Add all the ingredients in a high-speed blender and pulse until smooth.
2. Pour the smoothie into two glasses and serve immediately.

Nutrition : Calories 132; Total Fat 11.7 g; Saturated Fat 2.2 g; Cholesterol 0 mg; Sodium 27 mg; Total Carbs 6.1 g; Fiber 4.5 g; Sugar 0.4 g; Protein 3.1 g

Raisins – Plume Smoothie (RPS)

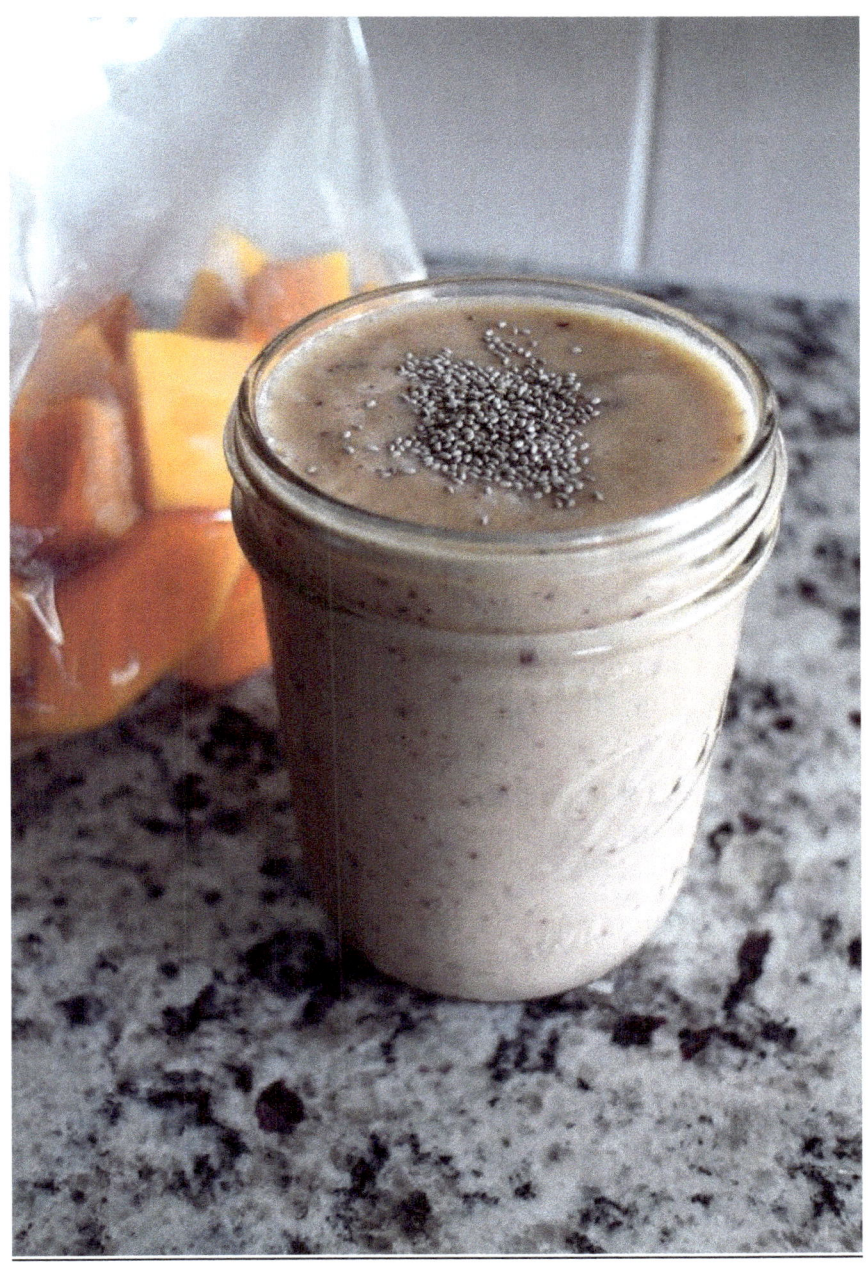

Preparation Time : 10 minutes

Cooking Time : 0 minutes

Servings : 1

Ingredients :

- 1 Teaspoon Raisins
- 2 Sweet Cherry
- 1 Skinned Black Plume
- 1 Cup Dr. Sebi's Stomach Calming Herbal Tea/ Cuachalate back powder,
- ¼ Coconut Water

Directions :

1. Flash 1 teaspoon of Raisin in warm water for 5 seconds and drain the water completely.

2. Rinse, cube Sweet Cherry and skinned black Plum

3. Get 1 cup of water boiled; put ¾ Dr. Sebi's Stomach Calming Herbal Tea for 10 – 15minutes.

4. If you are unable to get Dr. Sebi's Stomach Calming Herbal tea, you can alternatively, cook 1 teaspoon of powdered Cuachalate with 1 cup of water for 5 – 10 minutes, remove the extract and allow it to cool.

5. Pour all the ARPS items inside a blender and blend till you achieve a homogenous smoothie.

6. It is now okay, for you to enjoy the inevitable detox smoothie.

Nutrition : Calories: 150; Fat: 1.2 g; Carbohydrates: 79 g; Protein: 3.1 g

Nori Clove Smoothies (NCS)

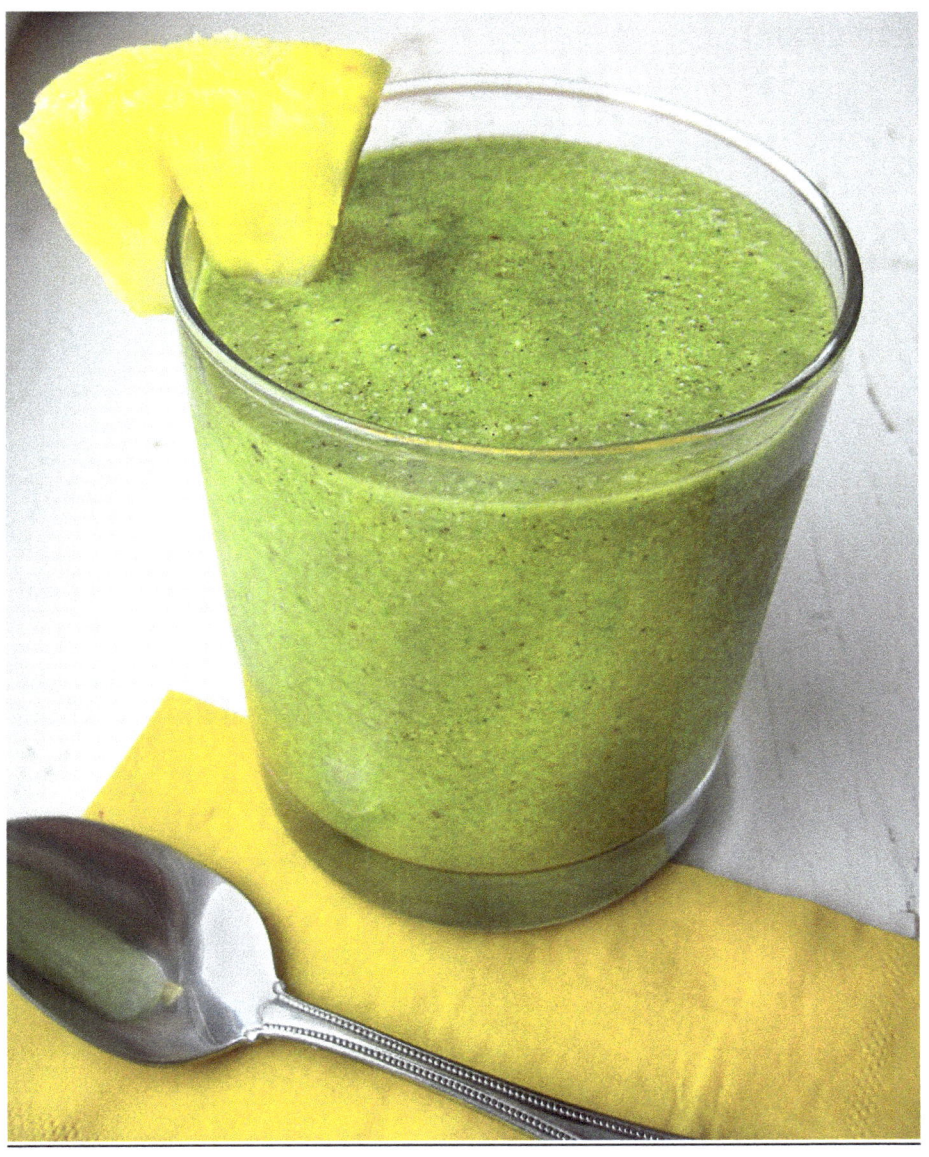

Preparation Time : 10 minutes

Cooking Time : 0 minutes

Servings : 1

Ingredients :

- ¼ Cup Fresh Nori
- 1 Cup Cubed Banana
- 1 Teaspoon Diced Onion or ¼ Teaspoon Powdered Onion
- ½ Teaspoon Clove
- 1 Cup Dr. Sebi Energy Booster
- 1 Tablespoon Agave Syrup

Directions :

1. Rinse ANCS Items with clean water.
2. Finely chop the onion to take one teaspoon and cut fresh Nori
3. Boil 1½ teaspoon with 2 cups of water, remove the particle, allow to cool, measure 1 cup of the tea extract
4. Pour all the items inside a blender with the tea extract and blend to achieve homogenous smoothies.
5. Transfer into a clean cup and have a nice time with a lovely body detox and energizer.

Nutrition : Calories: 78; Fat: 2.3 g; Carbohydrates: 5 g; Protein: 6 g

Brazil Lettuce Smoothies (BLS)

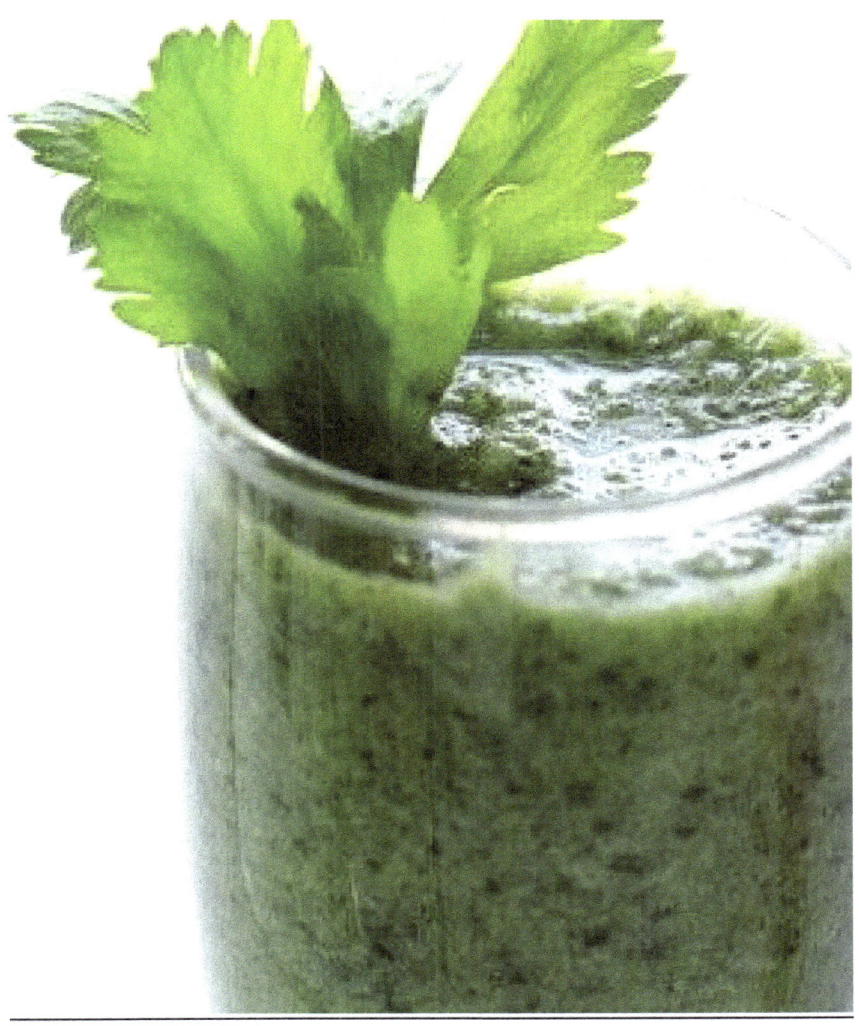

Preparation Time : 10 minutes

Cooking Time : 0 minutes

Servings : 1

Ingredients :

- 1 Cup Raspberries
- ½ Handful Romaine Lettuce
- ½ Cup Homemade Walnut Milk
- 2 Brazil Nuts
- ½ Large Grape with Seed
- 1 Cup Soft jelly Coconut Water
- Date Sugar to Taste

Directions :

1. In a clean bowl rinse, the vegetable with clean water.
2. Chop the Romaine Lettuce and cubed Raspberries and add other items into the blender and blend to achieve homogenous smoothies.
3. Serve your delicious medicinal detox.

Nutrition : Calories: 168; Fat: 4.5 g; Carbohydrates: 31.3 g; Sugar: 19.2 g; Protein: 3.6 g

Apple – Banana Smoothie (Abs)

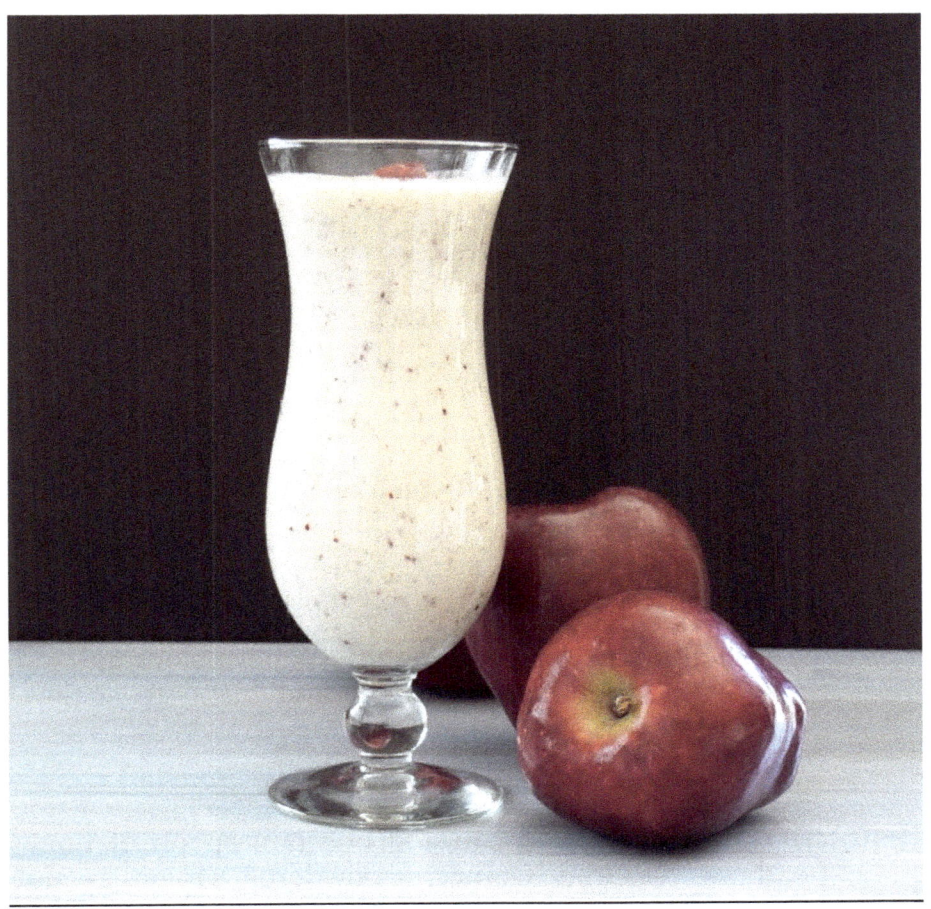

Preparation Time : 10 minutes

Cooking Time : 0 minutes

Servings : 1

Ingredients :

- I Cup Cubed Apple
- ½ Burro Banana
- ½ Cup Cubed Mango
- ½ Cup Cubed Watermelon
- ½ Teaspoon Powdered Onion
- 3 Tablespoon Key Lime Juice
- Date Sugar to Taste (If you like)

Directions :

1. In a clean bowl rinse, the vegetable with clean water.
2. Cubed Banana, Apple, Mango, Watermelon and add other items into the blender and blend to achieve homogenous smoothies.
3. Serve your delicious medicinal detox.
4. Alternatively, you can add one tablespoon of finely dices raw red Onion if powdered Onion is not available.

Nutrition : Calories: 99; Fat: 0.3g; Carbohydrates: 23 grams; Protein: 1.1 g

Ginger – Pear Smoothie (GPS)

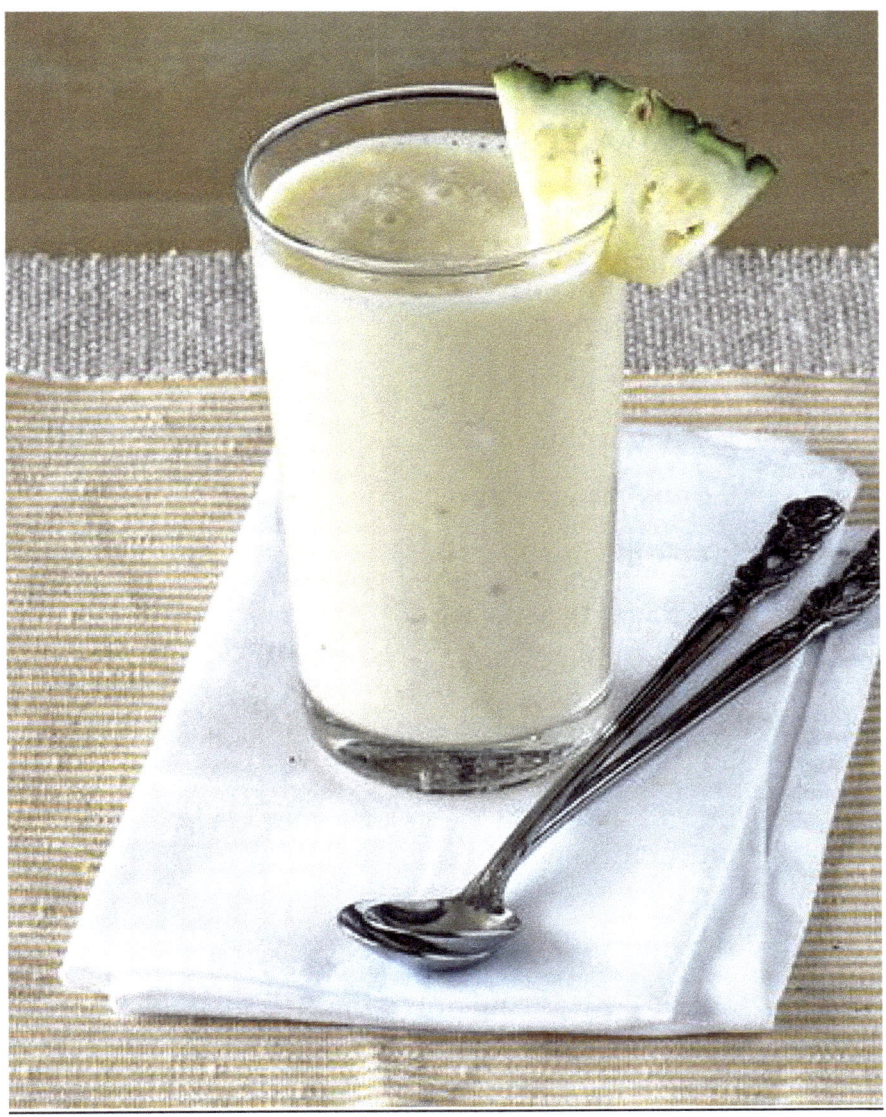

Preparation Time : 10 minutes

Cooking Time : 0 minutes

Servings : 1

Ingredients :

- 1 Big Pear with Seed and Cured
- ½ Avocado
- ¼ Handful Watercress
- ½ Sour Orange
- ½ Cup Ginger Tea
- ½ Cup Coconut Water
- ¼ Cup Spring Water
- 2 Tablespoon Agave Syrup
- Date Sugar to satisfaction

Directions :

1. Firstly boil 1 cup of Ginger Tea, cover the cup and allow it cool to room temperature.

2. Pour all the AGPS Items into your clean blender and homogenize them to smooth fluid.

3. You have just prepared yourself a wonderful Detox Romaine Smoothie.

Nutrition : Calories: 101; Protein: 1 g; Carbs: 27 g; Fiber: 6 g

Cantaloupe – Amaranth Smoothie (CAS)

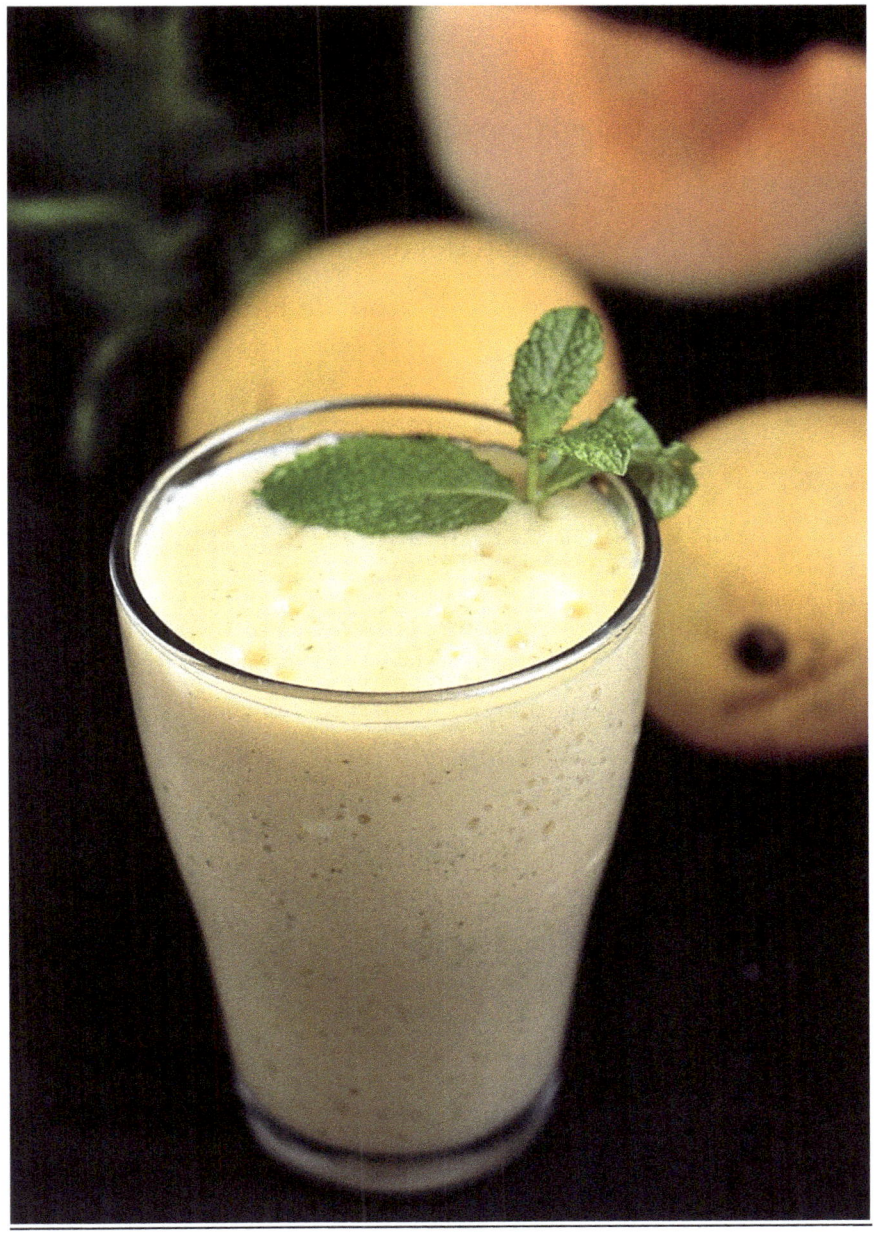

Preparation Time : 10 minutes

Cooking Time : 0 minutes

Servings : 1

Ingredients :

- ½ Cup Cubed Cantaloupe
- ¼ Handful Green Amaranth
- ½ Cup Homemade Hemp Milk
- ¼ Teaspoon Dr. Sebi's Bromide Plus Powder
- 1 Cup Coconut Water
- 1 Teaspoon Agave Syrup

Directions :

1. You will have to rinse all the ACAS items with clean water.

2. Chop green Amaranth, cubed Cantaloupe, transfer all into a blender and blend to achieve homogenous smoothie.

3. Pour into a clean cup; add Agave syrup and homemade Hemp Milk.

4. Stir them together and drink.

Nutrition : Calories: 55; Fiber: 1.5 g; Carbohydrates: 8 mg

Garbanzo Squash Smoothie (GSS)

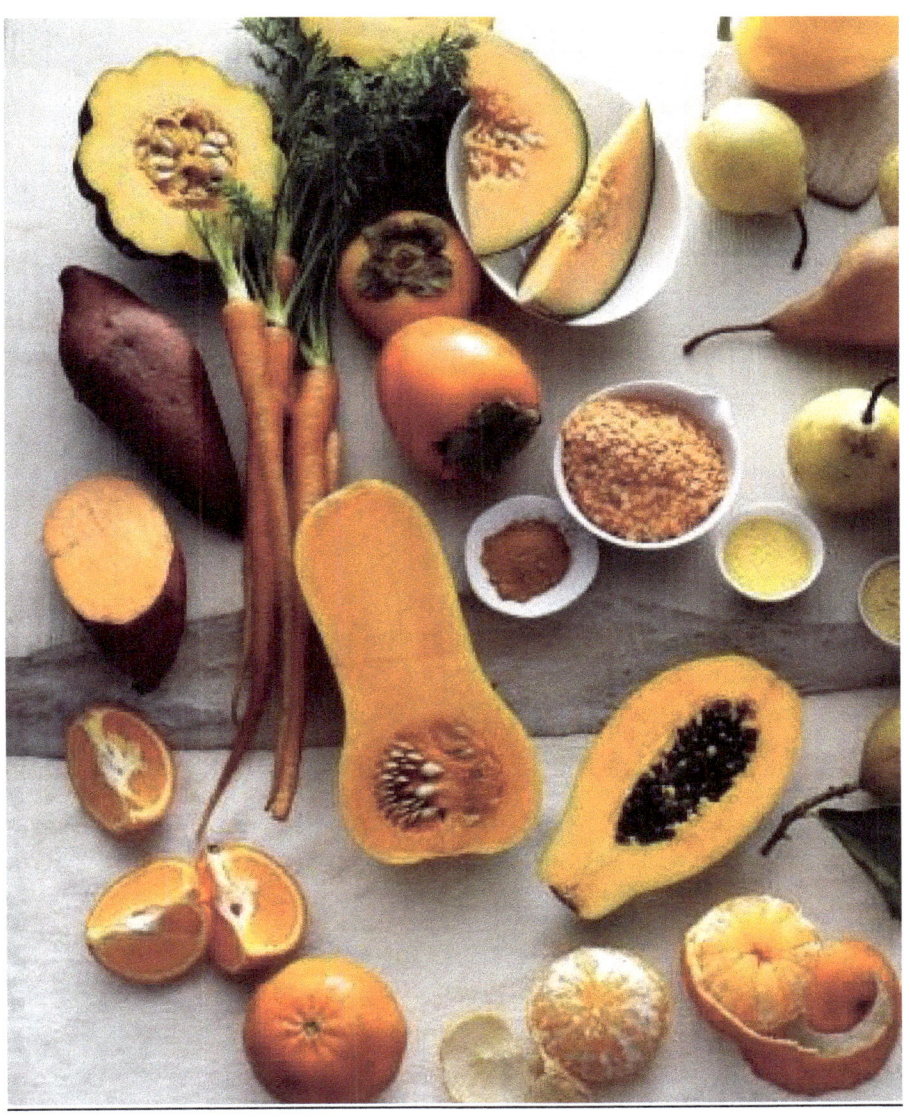

Preparation Time : 10 minutes

Cooking Time : 0 minutes

Servings : 1

Ingredients :

- 1 Large Cubed Apple
- 1 Fresh Tomatoes
- 1 Tablespoon Finely Chopped Fresh Onion or ¼ Teaspoon Powdered Onion
- ¼ Cup Boiled Garbanzo Bean
- ½ Cup Coconut Milk
- ¼ Cubed Mexican Squash Chayote
- 1 Cup Energy Booster Tea

Directions :

1. You will need to rinse the AGSS items with clean water.
2. Boil 1½ Dr. Sebi's Energy Booster Tea with 2 cups of clean water. Filter the extract, measure 1 cup and allow it to cool.
3. Cook Garbanzo Bean, drain the water and allow it to cool.
4. Pour all the AGSS items into a high-speed blender and blend to achieve homogenous smoothie.
5. You may add Date Sugar.
6. Serve your amazing smoothie and drink.

Nutrition : Calories: 82; Carbs: 22 g; Protein: 2 g; Fiber: 7 g

Strawberry – Orange Smoothies (SOS)

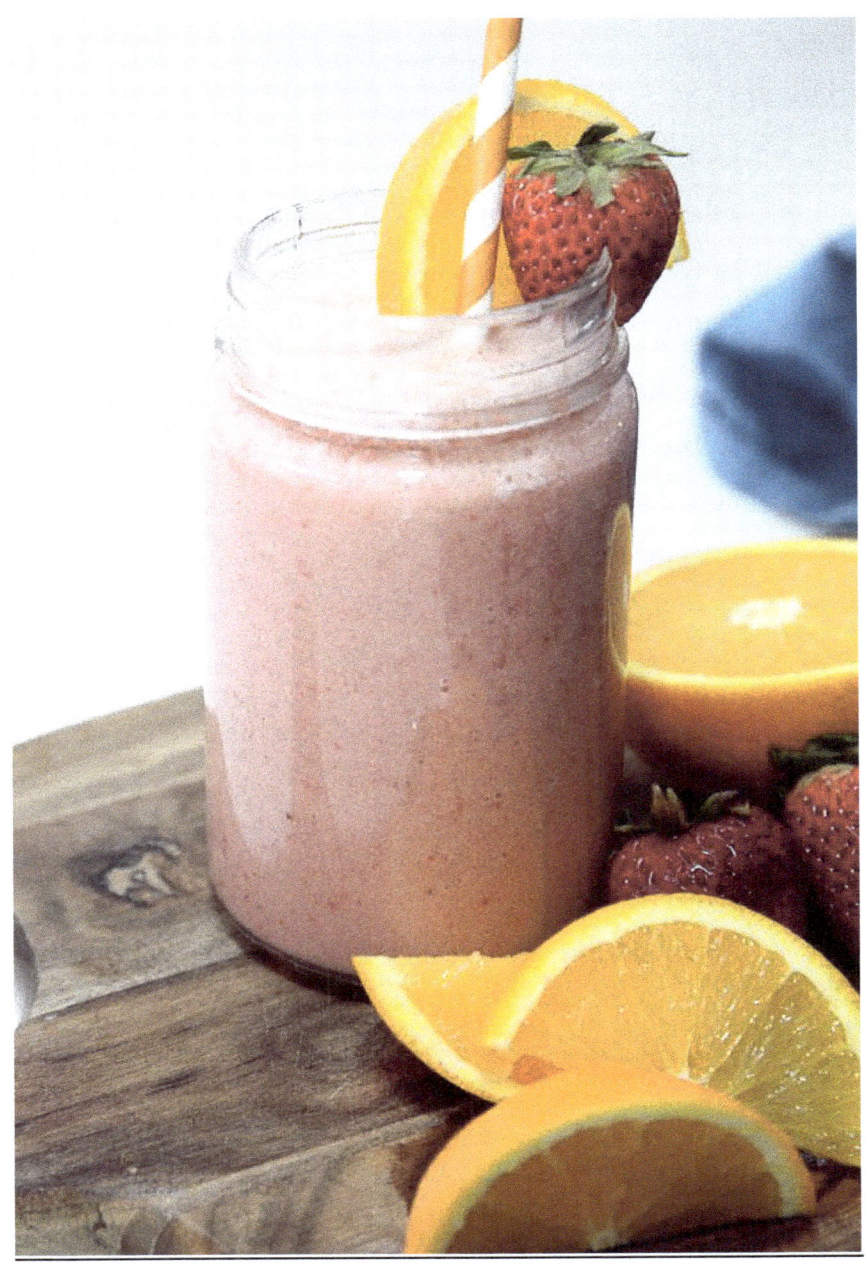

Preparation Time : 10 minutes

Cooking Time : 0 minutes

Servings : 1

Ingredients :

- 1 Cup Diced Strawberries
- 1 Removed Back of Seville Orange
- ¼ Cup Cubed Cucumber
- ¼ Cup Romaine Lettuce
- ½ Kelp
- ½ Burro Banana
- 1 Cup Soft Jelly Coconut Water
- ½ Cup Water
- Date Sugar.

Directions :

1. Use clean water to rinse all the vegetable items of ASOS into a clean bowl.

2. Chop Romaine Lettuce; dice Strawberry, Cucumber, and Banana; remove the back of Seville Orange and divide into four.

3. Transfer all the ASOS items inside a clean blender and blend to achieve a homogenous smoothie.

4. Pour into a clean big cup and fortify your body with a palatable detox.

Nutrition : Calories 298; Calories from Fat 9; Fat 1g; Cholesterol 2mg; Sodium 73mg; Potassium 998mg; Carbohydrates 68g; Fiber 7g; Sugar 50g

Tamarind – Pear Smoothie (TPS)

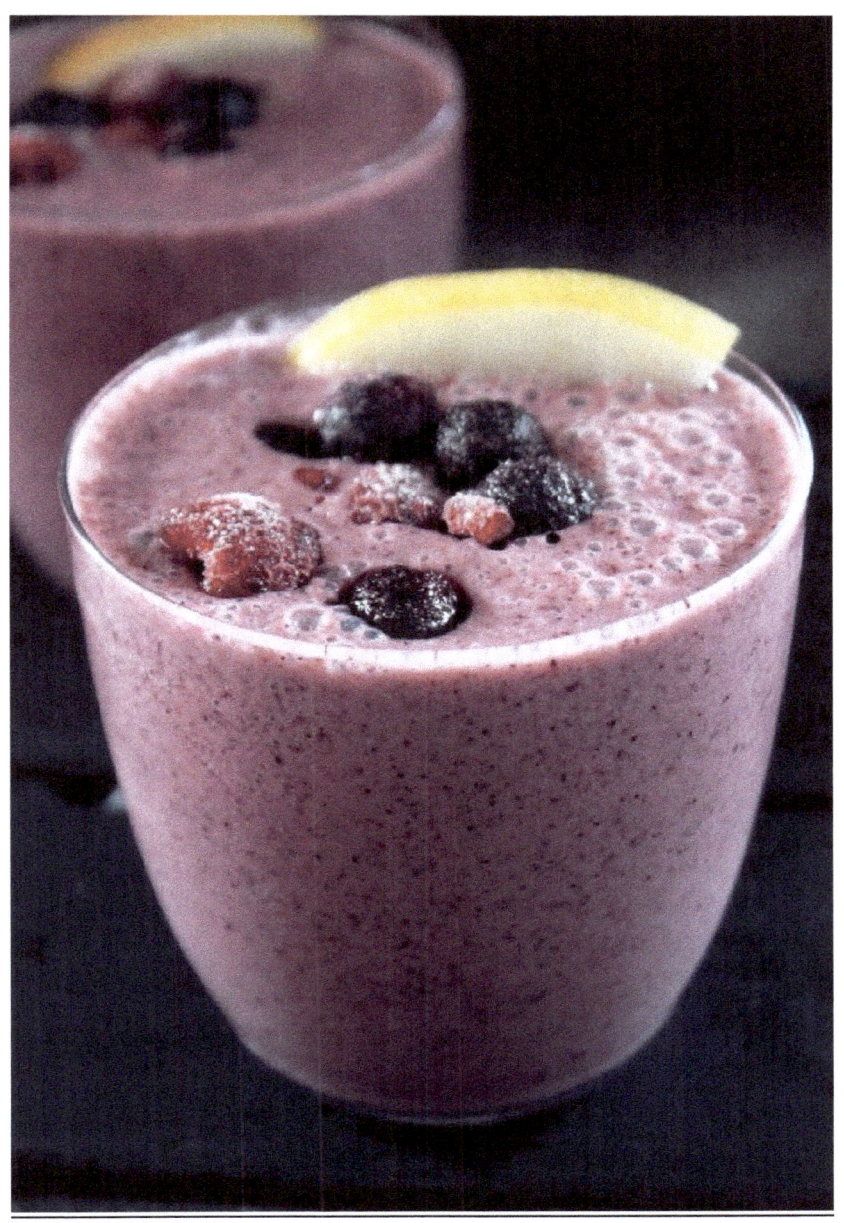

Preparation Time : 10 minutes

Cooking Time : 0 minutes

Servings : 1

Ingredients :

- ½ Burro Banana
- ½ Cup Watermelon
- 1 Raspberries
- 1 Prickly Pear
- 1 Grape with Seed
- 3 Tamarind
- ½ Medium Cucumber
- 1 Cup Coconut Water
- ½ Cup Distilled Water

Directions :

1. Use clean water to rinse all the ATPS items.

2. Remove the pod of Tamarind and collect the edible part around the seed into a container.

3. If you must use the seeds then you have to boil the seed for 15mins and add to the Tamarind edible part in the container.

4. Cubed all other vegetable fruits and transfer all the items into a high-speed blender and blend to achieve homogenous smoothie.

Nutrition : Calories: 199; Carbohydrates: 47 g; Fat: 1g; Protein: 6g

Currant Elderberry Smoothie (CES)

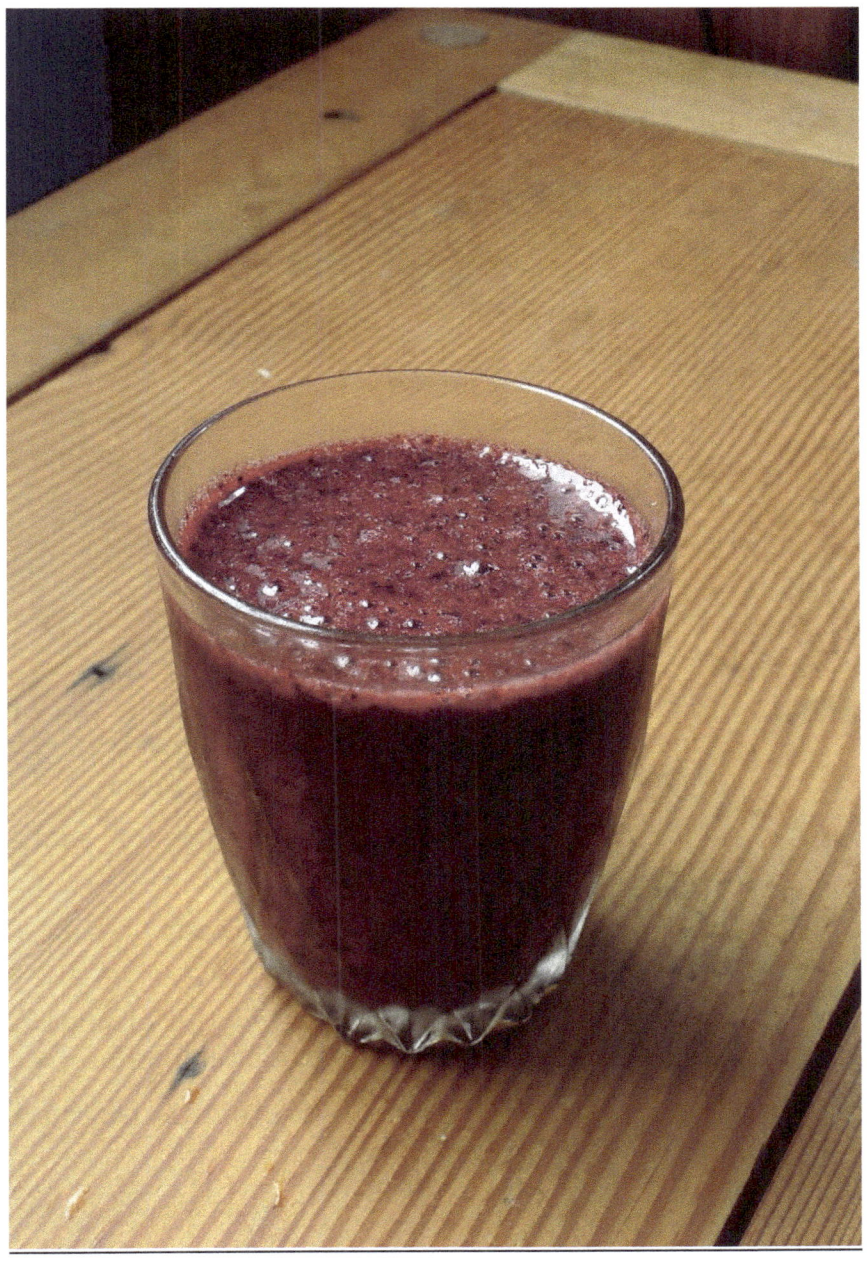

Preparation Time : 10 minutes

Cooking Time : 0 minutes

Servings : 1

Ingredients :

- ¼ Cup Cubed Elderberry
- 1 Sour Cherry
- 2 Currant
- 1 Cubed Burro Banana
- 1 Fig
- 1Cup 4 Bay Leaves Tea
- 1 Cup Energy Booster Tea
- Date Sugar to your satisfaction

Directions :

1. Use clean water to rinse all the ACES items

2. Initially boil ¾ Teaspoon of Energy Booster Tea with 2 cups of water on a heat source and allow boiling for 10 minutes.

3. Add 4 Bay leaves and boil together for another 4minutes.

4. Drain the Tea extract into a clean big cup and allow it to cool.

5. Transfer all the items into a high-speed blender and blend till you achieve a homogenous smoothie.

6. Pour the palatable medicinal smoothie into a clean cup and drink.

Nutrition : Calories: 63; Fat: 0.22g; Sodium: 1.1mg; Carbohydrates: 15.5g; Fiber: 4.8g; Sugars: 8.25g; Protein: 1.6g

Sweet Dream Strawberry Smoothie

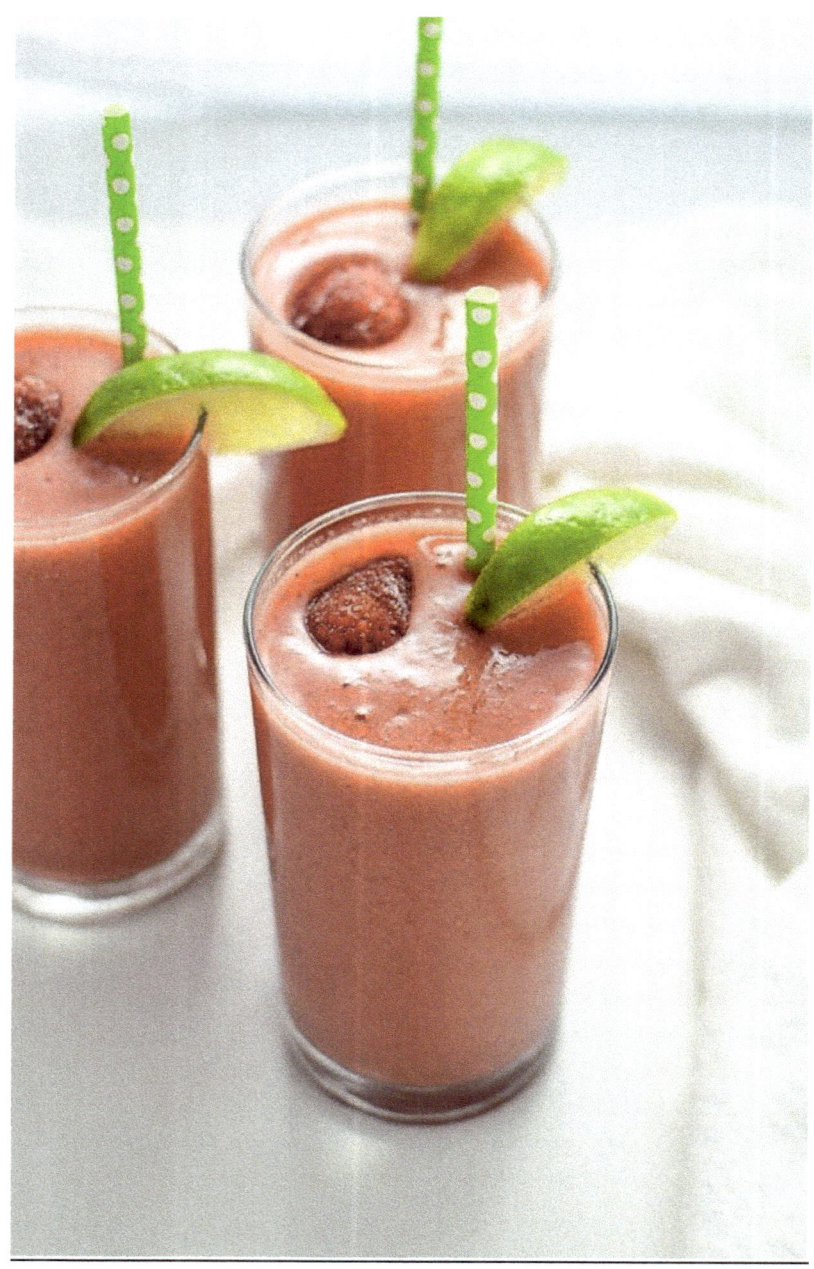

Preparation Time :1 5 minutes

Cooking Time : 0

Servings : 1

Ingredients :

- 5 Strawberries
- 3 Dates – Pits eliminated
- 2 Burro Bananas or small bananas
- Spring Water for 32 fluid ounces of smoothie

Directions :

1. Strip off skin of the bananas.
2. Wash the dates and strawberries.
3. Include bananas, dates, and strawberries to a blender container.
4. Include a couple of water and blend.
5. Keep on including adequate water to persuade up to be 32 oz. of smoothie.

Nutrition : Calories: 282; Fat: 11g; Carbohydrates: 4g; Protein: 7g

Alkaline Green Ginger and Banana Cleansing Smoothie

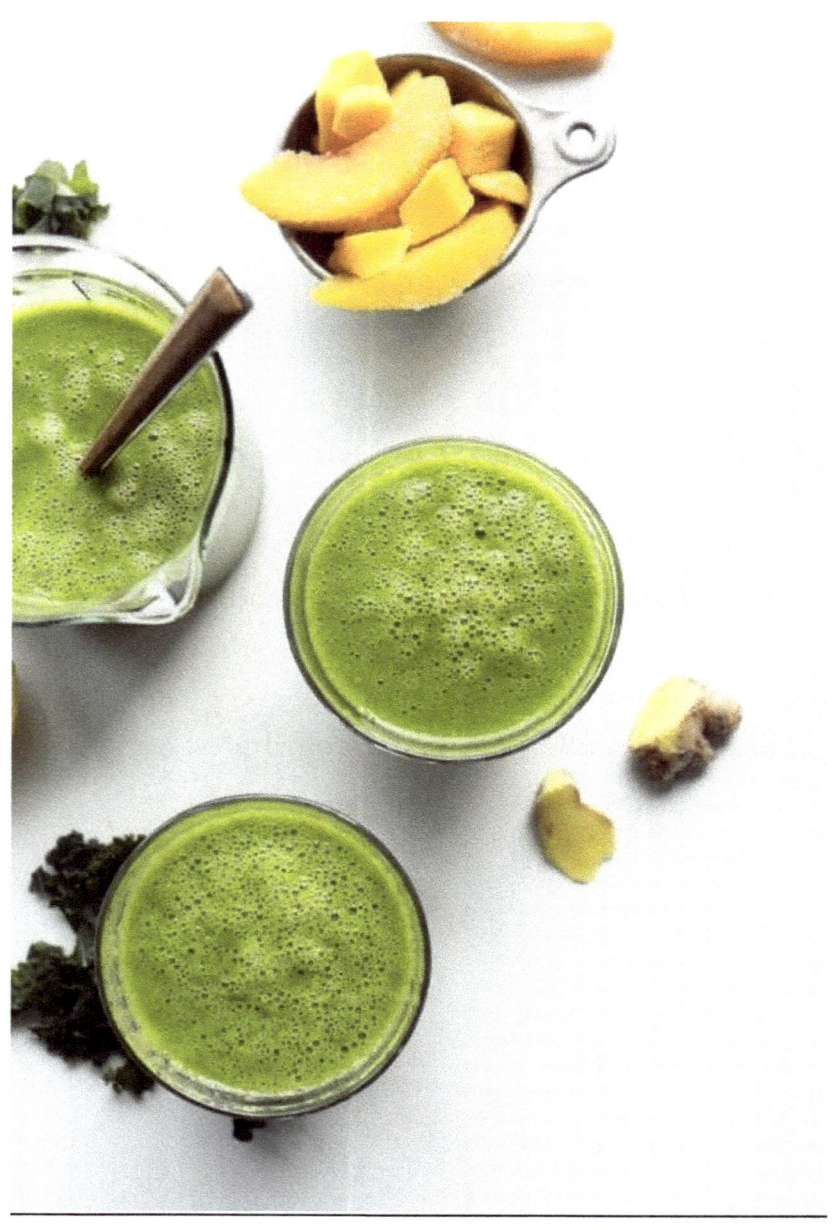

Preparation Time : 15 minutes

Cooking Time : 0

Servings : 1

Ingredients :

- One handful of kale
- one banana, frozen
- Two cups of hemp seed milk
- One inch of ginger, finely minced
- Half cup of chopped strawberries, frozen
- 1 tablespoon of agave or your preferred sweetener

Directions :

1. Mix all the Ingredients in a blender and mix on high speed.
2. Allow it to blend evenly.
3. Pour into a pitcher with a few decorative straws and voila you are one happy camper.
4. *Enjoy!*

Nutrition : Calories: 350; Fat: 4g; Carbohydrates: 52g; Protein: 16g

Orange Mixed Detox Smoothie

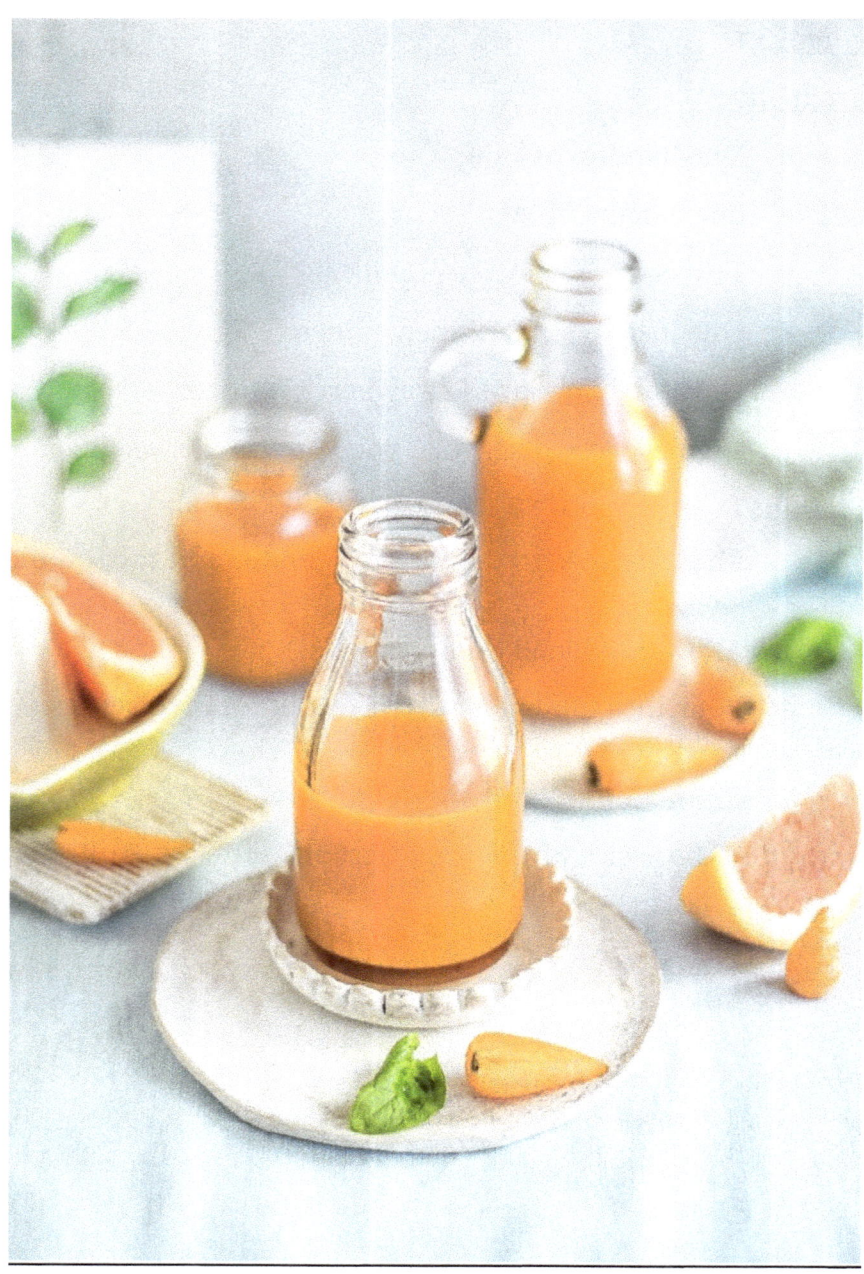

Preparation Time : 15 minutes

Cooking Time : 0

Servings : 1

Ingredients :

- One cup of vegies (Amaranth, Dandelion, Lettuce or Watercress)
- Half avocado
- One cup of tender-jelly coconut water
- One seville orange
- Juice of one key lime
- One tablespoon of bromide plus powder

Directions :

1. Peel and cut the Seville orange in chunks.
2. *Mix all the Ingredients collectively in a high-speed blender until done.*

Nutrition : Calories: 71; Fat: 1g; Carbohydrates: 12g; Protein: 2g

Cucumber Toxin Flush Smoothie

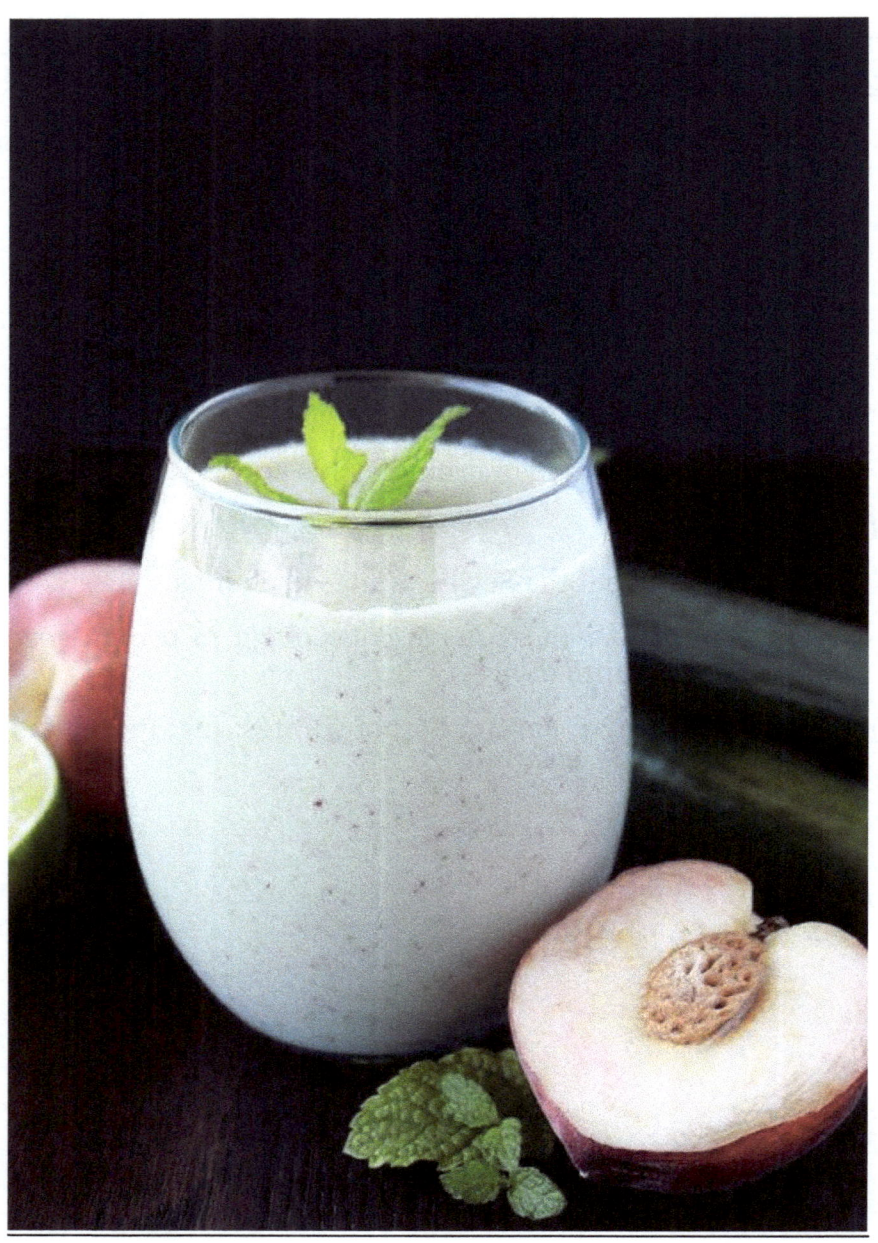

Preparation Time : 15 minutes

Cooking Time : 0

Servings : 1

Ingredients :

- 1 Cucumber
- 1 Key Lime
- 1 cup of watermelon (seeded), cubed

Directions :

1. Mix all the above Ingredients in a high-speed blender.
2. Considering that watermelon and cucumbers are largely water, you may not want to add any extra, however you can so if you want.
3. Juice the key lime and add into your smoothie.
4. *Enjoy!*

Nutrition : Calories: 219; Fat: 4g; Carbohydrates: 48g; Protein: 5g

Apple Blueberry Smoothie

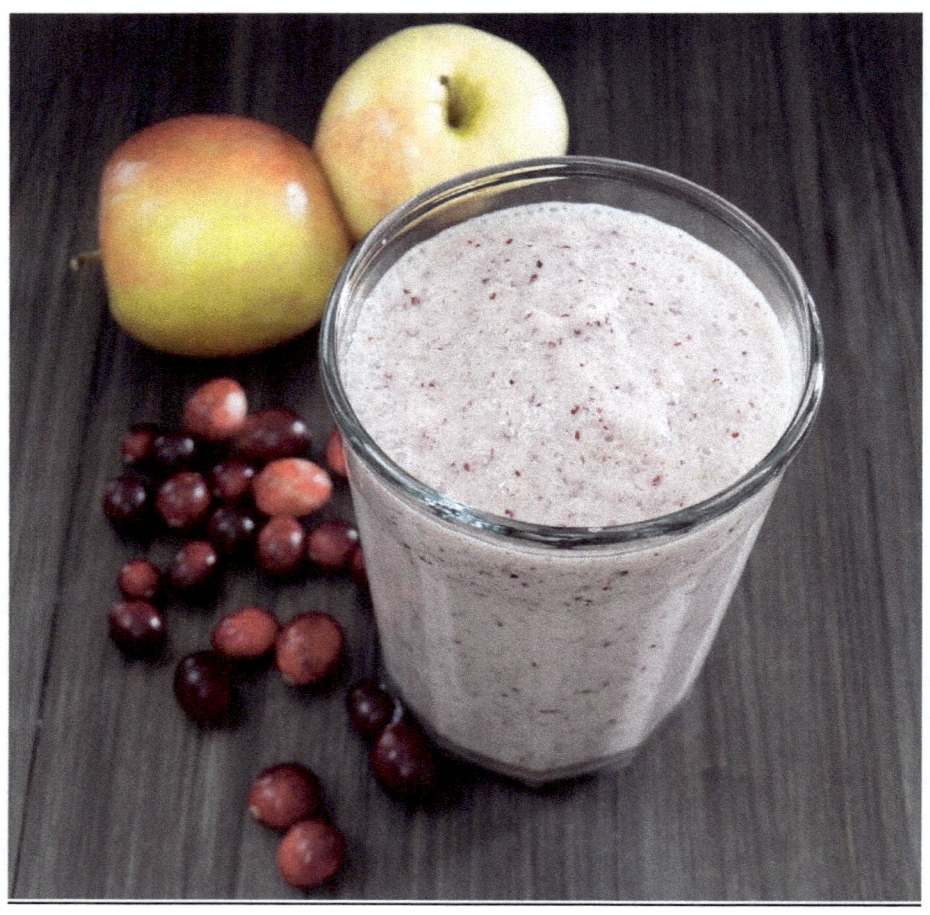

Preparation Time : 15 minutes

Cooking Time : 0

Servings : 1

Ingredients :

- Half apple
- One Date
- Half cup of blueberries
- Half cup of sparkling callaloo
- One tablespoon of hemp seeds
- One tablespoon of sesame seeds
- Two cups of sparkling soft-jelly coconut water
- Half of tablespoon of bromide plus powder

Directions :

1. *Mix all of the Ingredients in a high-speed blender and enjoy!*

Nutrition : Calories: 167.4; Fat: 6.4g; Carbohydrates: 22.5g; Protein: 6.7g

Lemon Rooibos Iced Tea

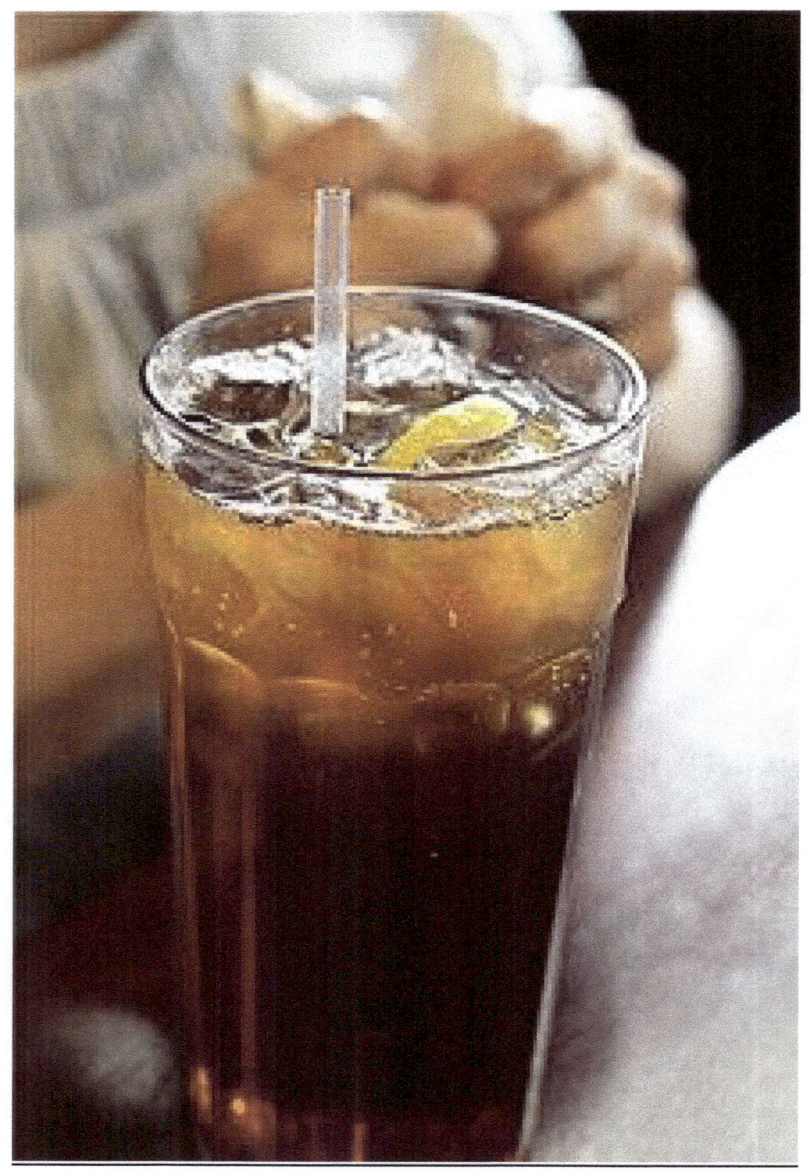

Preparation Time : 10 minutes

Cooking Time : 0 minute

Serving : 4

Ingredients :

- 4 bags natural, unflavored rooibos tea
- 4 cups boiling water
- 3 tablespoons freshly squeezed lemon juice
- 30–40 drops liquid stevia

Directions:

1. Situate tea bags into tea pot and pour the boiling water over the bags.

2. Set aside to room temperature, then refrigerate the tea until it is ice-cold.

3. Remove the tea bags. Squeeze them gently.

4. Add the lemon juice and liquid stevia to taste and stir until well mixed.

5. Serve immediately, preferably with ice cubes and some nice garnishes, like lemon wedges.

Nutrition : 70 Calories; 16g Carbohydrates; 1g Protein

Lemon Lavender Iced Tea

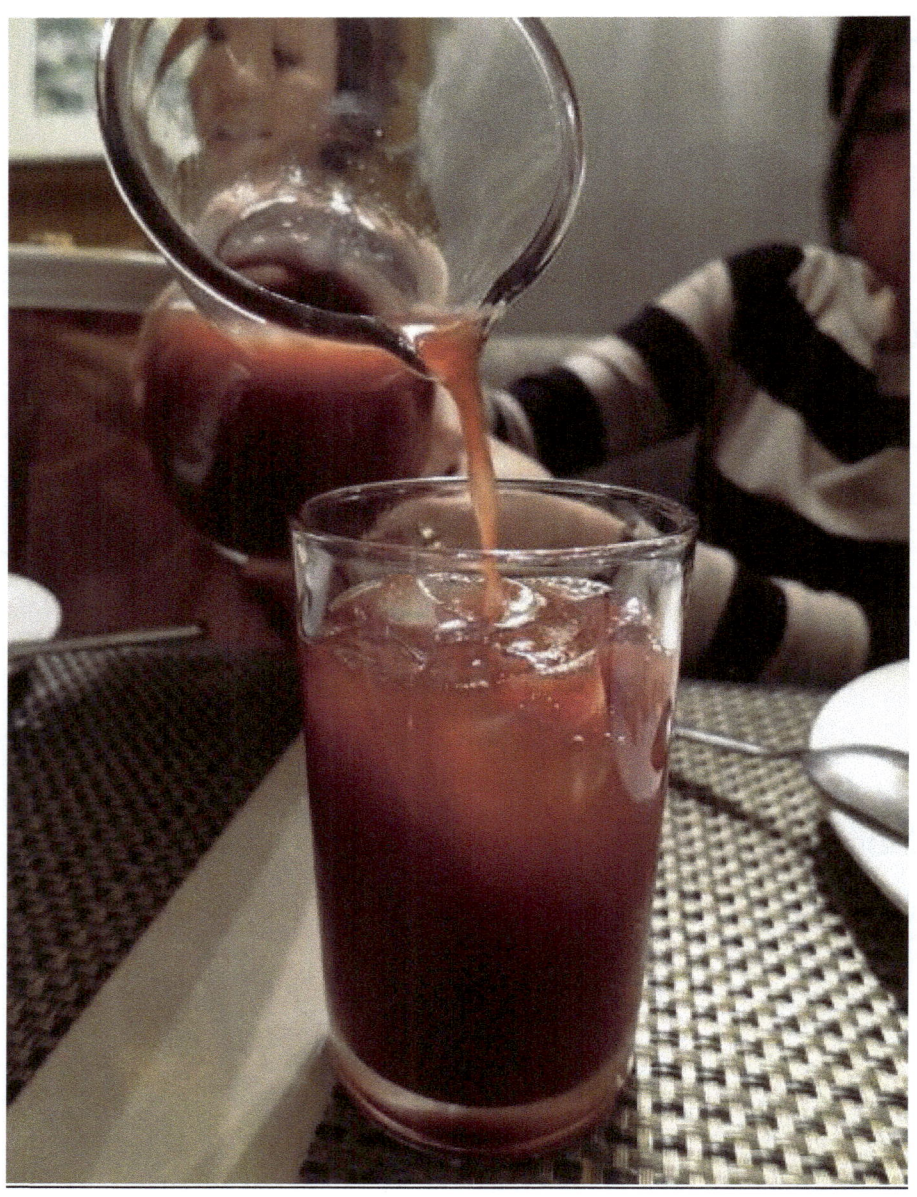

Preparation Time : 15minutes

Cooking Time : 0 minute

Serving : 4

Ingredients :

- 2 bags natural, unflavored rooibos tea
- 2 oz lemon chunks without peel and pith, seeds removed
- 1 teaspoon dried lavender blossoms placed in a tea ball
- 4 cups water, at room temperature
- 20–40 drops liquid stevia

Directions:

1. Place the tea bags, lemon chunks and the tightly-closed tea ball with the lavender blossoms in a 1.5 qt (1.5 l) pitcher.
2. Pour in the water.
3. Refrigerate overnight.
4. Remove the tea bags, lemon chunks and the tea ball with the lavender on the next day. Squeeze the tea bags gently to save as much liquid as possible.
5. Add liquid stevia to taste and stir until well mixed.
6. Serve immediately with ice cubes and lemon wedges.

Nutrition : 81 Calories; 12g Carbohydrates; 3g Protein

Cherry Vanilla Iced Tea

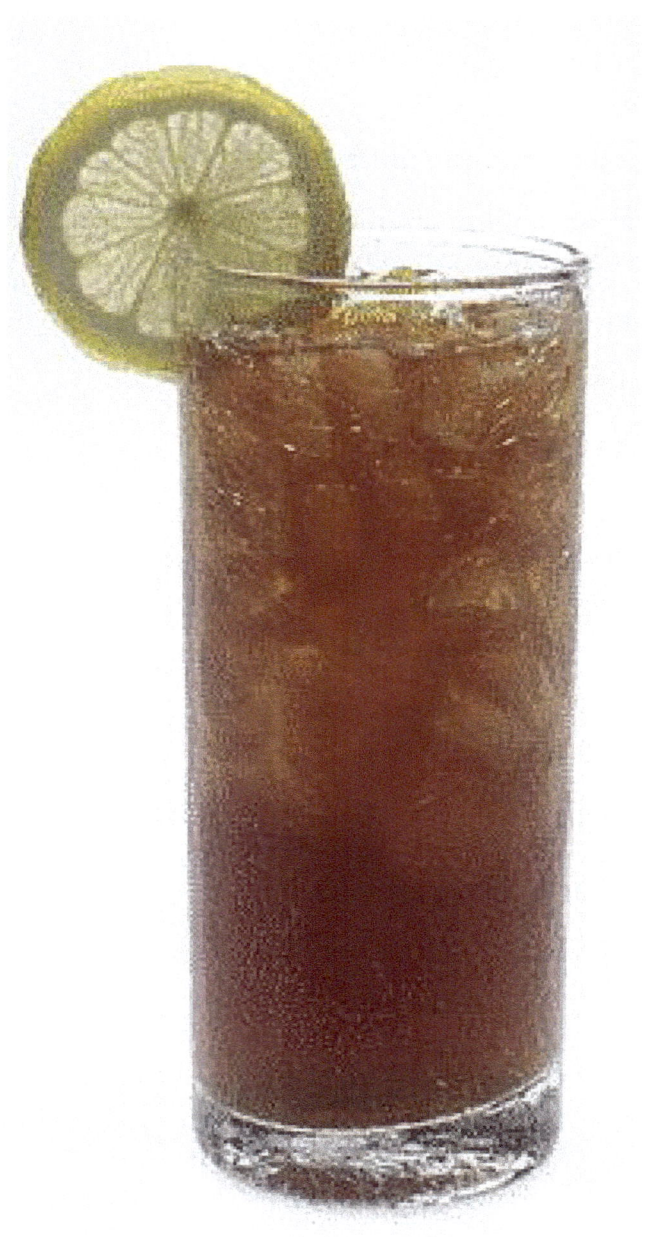

Preparation Time : 12 minutes

Cooking Time : 0 minute

Serving : 4

Ingredients :

- 4 bags natural, unflavored rooibos tea
- 4 cups boiling water
- 2 tablespoons freshly squeezed lime juice
- 1–2 tablespoons cherry flavoring
- 30–40 drops (or to taste) liquid vanilla stevia

Directions:

1. Place tea bags into tea pot and pour the boiling water over the bags.
2. Put aside the tea cool down first, then refrigerate the tea until it is ice-cold.
3. Remove the tea bags. Squeeze them lightly.
4. Add the lime juice, cherry flavoring and the vanilla stevia and stir until well mixed.
5. Serve immediately, preferably with ice cubes and some nice garnishes like lime wedges and fresh cherries.

Nutrition : 89 Calories; 14g Carbohydrates; 2g Protein

Elegant Blueberry Rose Water Iced Tea

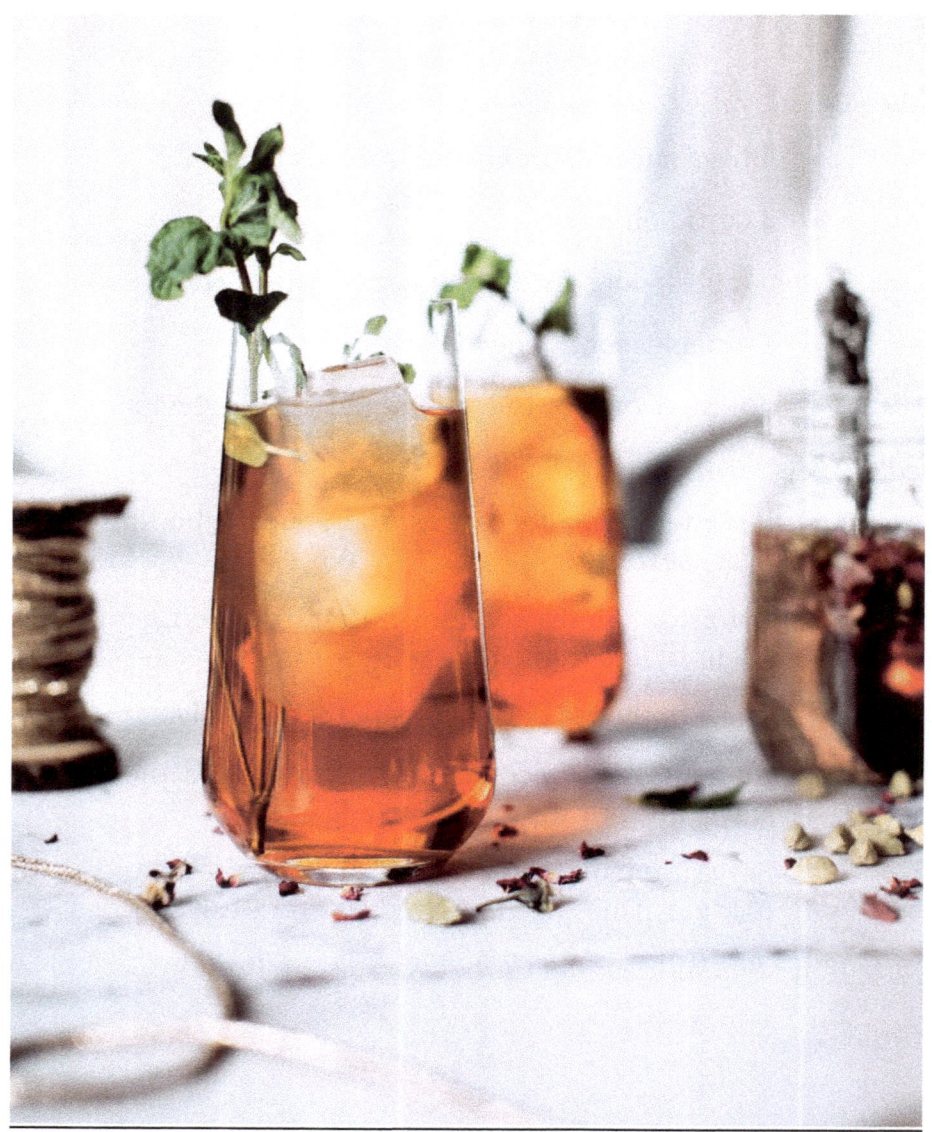

Preparation Time : 12 minutes

Cooking Time : 0 minute

Serving : 4

Ingredients :

- 2 bags herbal blueberry tea
- 4 cups boiling water
- 20 drops liquid stevia
- 1 tablespoon rose water

Directions:

1. Position tea bags into tea pot and pour the boiling water over the bags.

2. Allow tea cool down first, then refrigerate the tea until it is ice-cold.

3. Remove the tea bags. Press them gently.

4. Add the liquid stevia and the rose water and stir until well mixed.

5. Serve immediately, preferably with ice cubes and some nice garnishes, like fresh blueberries or natural rose petals

Nutrition : 75 Calories; 10g Carbohydrates; 2g Protein

Melba Iced Tea

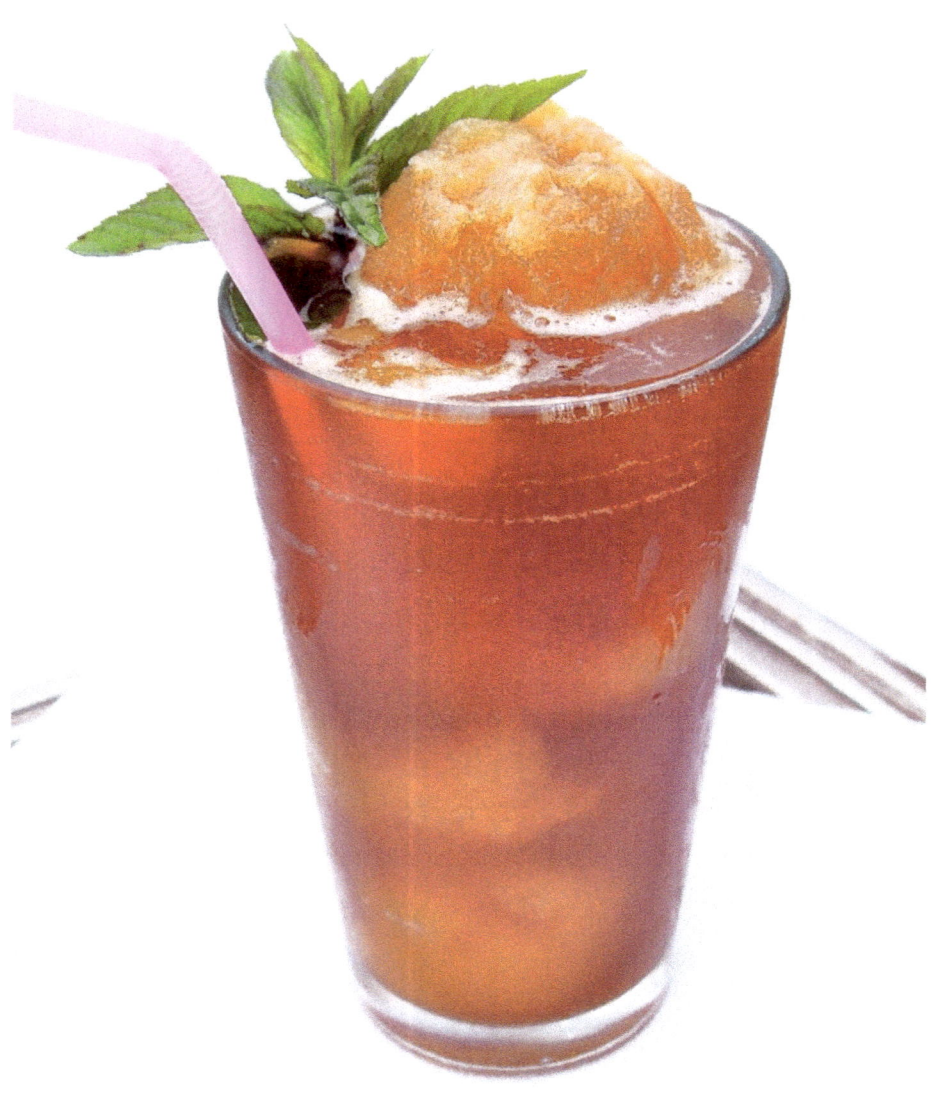

Preparation Time : 10 minutes

Cooking Time : 0 minute

Serving : 4

Ingredients :

- 1 bag herbal raspberry tea
- 1 bag herbal peach tea
- 4 cups boiling water
- 10 drops liquid peach stevia
- 20–40 drops (or to taste) liquid vanilla stevia

Directions :

1. Pour the boiling water over the tea bags.
2. Leave tea cool down on room temperature, then refrigerate the tea until it is ice-cold.
3. Remove the tea bags. Press lightly.
4. Add the peach stevia and stir until well mixed.
5. Add vanilla stevia to taste and stir until well mixed.
6. Serve immediately, preferably with ice cubes and some nice garnishes, like vanilla bean, fresh raspberries or peach slices.

Nutrition : 81 Calories; 14g Carbohydrates; 4g Protein

Merry Raspberry Cherry Iced Tea

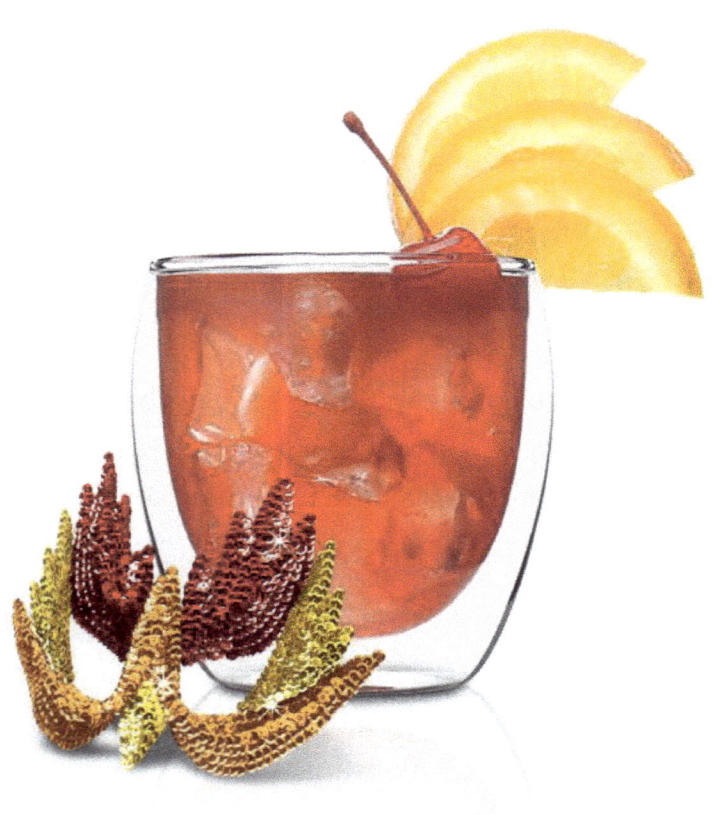

Preparation Time : 11 minutes

Cooking Time : 0 minute

Serving : 4

Ingredients :

- 2 bags herbal raspberry tea

- 4 cups boiling water

- 1 teaspoon stevia-sweetened cherry-flavored drink mix

- 1 teaspoon freshly squeezed lime juice

- 10–20 drops (or to taste) liquid stevia

Directions :

1. Put the tea bags into tea pot and fill in boiling water over the bags.

2. Let the tea cool down first to room temperature, then chill until it is ice-cold.

3. Discard tea bags. Squeeze them.

4. Add the cherry-flavored drink mix and the lime juice and stir until the drink mix is dissolved.

5. Add liquid stevia to taste and stir until well mixed.

6. Serve immediately, preferably with ice cubes or crushed ice and some nice garnishes, like fresh raspberries and cherries.

Nutrition : 82 Calories; 11g Carbohydrates; 4g Protein

Vanilla Kissed Peach Iced Tea

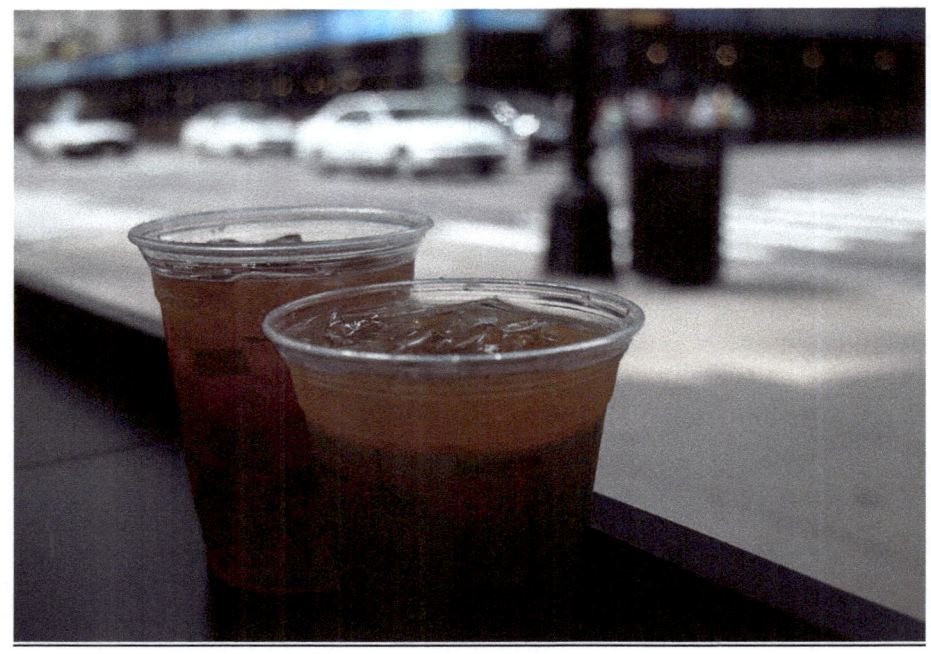

Preparation Time : 13 minutes

Cooking Time : 0 minute

Serving : 4

Ingredients :

- 2 bags herbal peach tea
- 4 cups boiling water
- 1 teaspoon vanilla extract
- 1 teaspoon freshly squeezed lemon juice
- 30–40 drops (or to taste) liquid stevia

Directions:

1. Soak tea bags over boiling water.
2. Allow to cool down on room temperature, then refrigerate the tea until it is ice-cold.
3. Remove and press tea bags.
4. Add the vanilla extract and the lemon juice and stir until well mixed.
5. Add liquid stevia to taste and stir until well mixed.
6. Serve immediately, preferably with ice cubes and some nice garnishes, like peach slices.

Nutrition : 88 Calories; 14g Carbohydrates; 3g Protein

Xtreme Berried Iced Tea

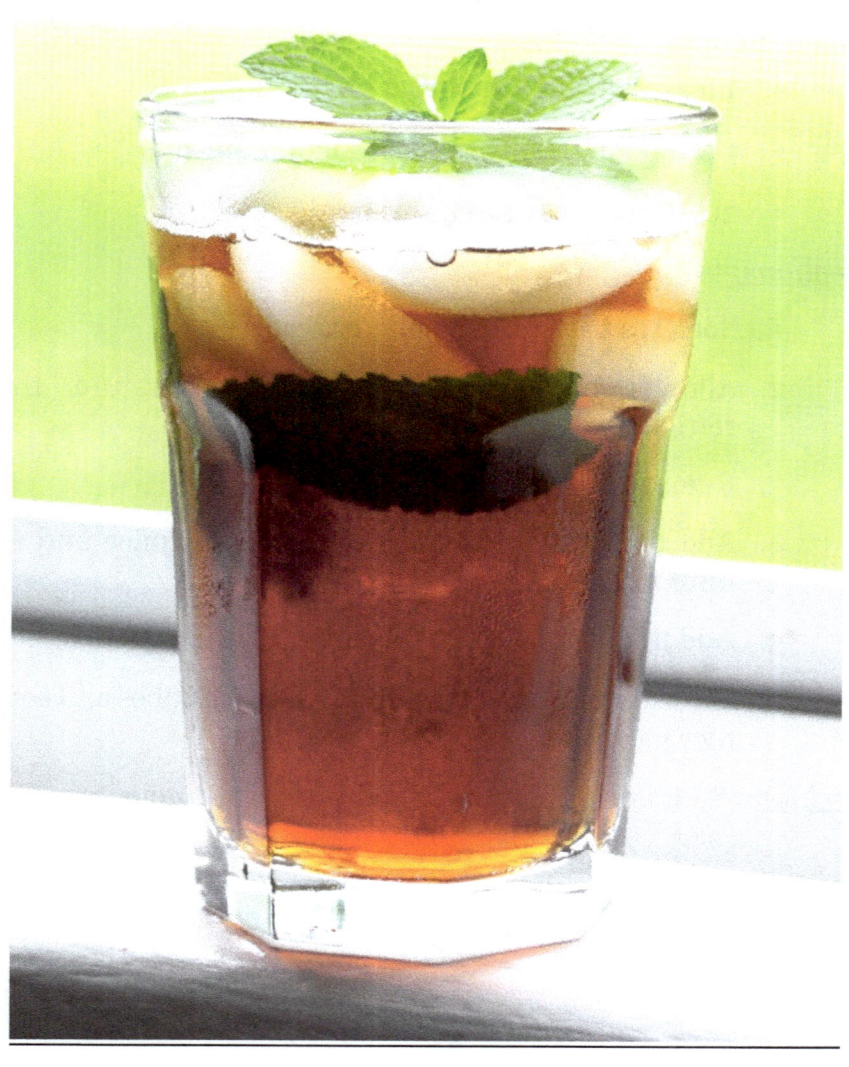

Preparation Time : 10 minutes

Cooking Time : 0 minute

Serving : 4

Ingredients :

- 2 bags herbal Wild Berry Tea
- 4 cups = 950 ml boiling water
- 2 teaspoons freshly squeezed lime juice
- 40 drops berry-flavored liquid stevia
- 10 drops (or to taste) liquid stevia

Directions:

1. Submerge tea bags into boiling water.
2. Set aside to cool down, then refrigerate the tea until it is ice- cold.
3. Pull out tea bags. Squeeze.
4. Add the lime juice and the berry stevia and stir until well mixed.
5. Add liquid stevia to taste and stir until well mixed.
6. Serve immediately.

Nutrition : 76 Calories; 14g Carbohydrates; 4g Protein

Refreshingly Peppermint Iced Tea

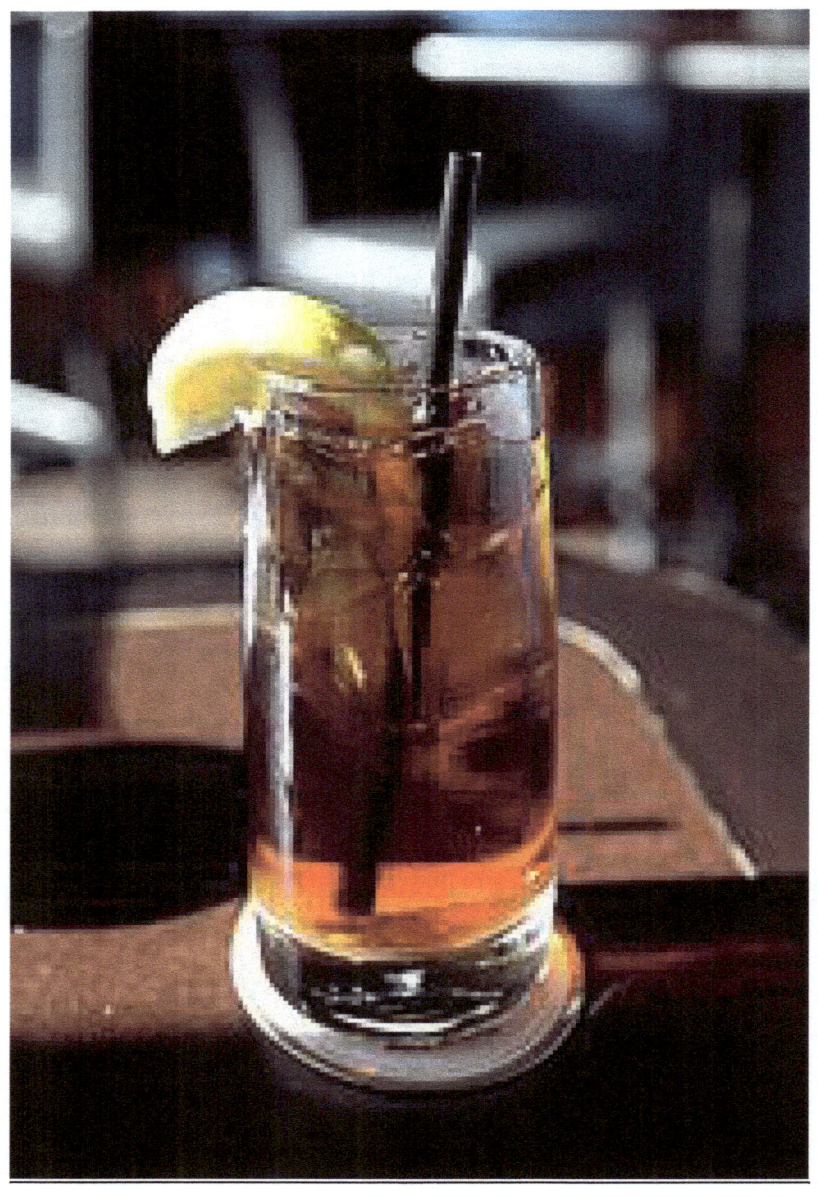

Preparation Time : 15 minutes

Cooking Time : 0 minute

Serving : 5

Ingredients :

- 4 bags peppermint tea
- 4 cups = 950 ml boiling water
- 2 teaspoons stevia-sweetened lime-flavored drink mix
- 1 cup = 240 ml ice-cold sparkling water

Directions:

1. Immerse tea bags on boiling water.
2. Set aside before cooling until it is ice-cold.
3. Take out tea bags then press.
4. Add the lime-flavored drink mix and stir until it is properly dissolved.
5. Add the sparkling water and stir very gently.
6. Serve immediately, preferably with ice cubes, mint leaves and lime wedges.

Nutrition : 78 Calories; 17g Carbohydrates; 4g Protein

Lemongrass Mint Iced Tea

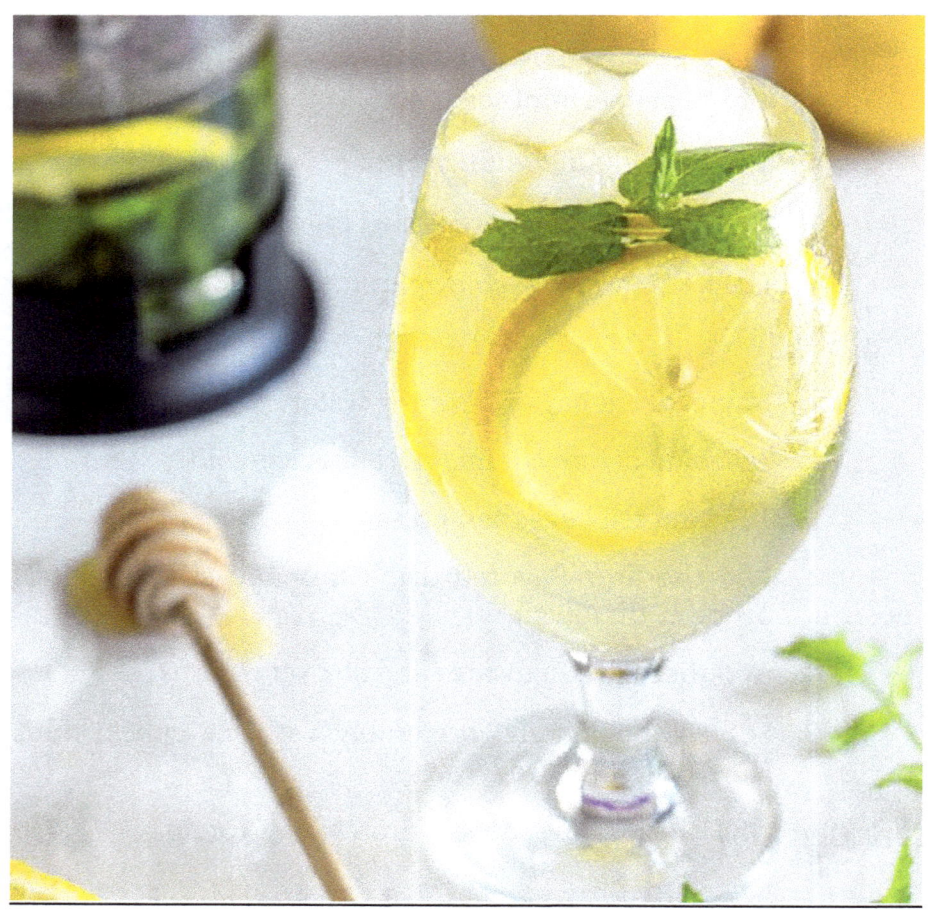

Preparation Time : 12 minutes

Cooking Time : 0 minute

Serving : 4

Ingredients :

- 1 stalk lemongrass, chopped in 1-inch
- 1/2 cup chopped, loosely packed mint sprigs
- 4 cups boiling water

Directions:

1. Put the lemongrass and the mint into tea pot and pour the boiling water over them.

2. Let cool down first to room temperature, then refrigerate until the tea is ice-cold.

3. Filter out the lemongrass and the mint.

4. Add liquid vanilla stevia to taste if you prefer some sweetness and stir until well mixed.

5. Serve immediately, preferably with ice cubes and some nice garnishes, like mint sprigs and lemongrass stalks.

Nutrition : 89 Calories; 17g Carbohydrates; 5g Protein

Spiced Tea

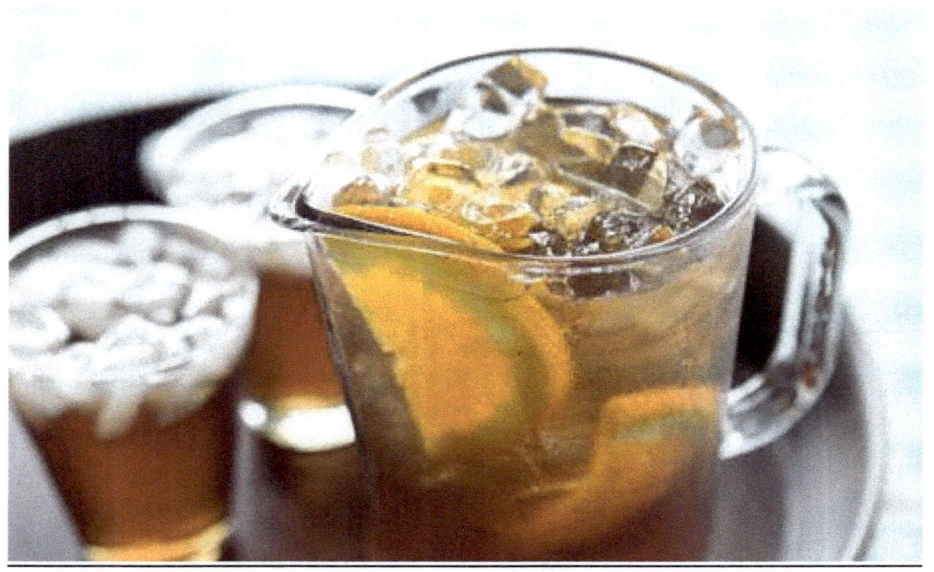

Preparation Time : 8 minutes

Cooking Time : 0 minute

Serving : 4

Ingredients :

- 2 bags Bengal Spice tea
- 2 teaspoons freshly squeezed lemon juice
- 1 packet zero-carb vanilla stevia
- 1 packet zero-carb stevia
- 4 cups boiling water

Directions:

1. Put the tea bags, lemon juice and the both stevia into tea pot.
2. Pour in the boiling water.
3. Put aside to cool over room temperature, then refrigerate.
4. Pull away tea bags then squeeze it.
5. Stir gently.
6. Serve immediately, preferably with ice cubes or crushed ice and some lemon wedges or slices.

Nutrition : 91 Calories; 16g Carbohydrates; 1g Protein

Infused Pumpkin Spice Latte

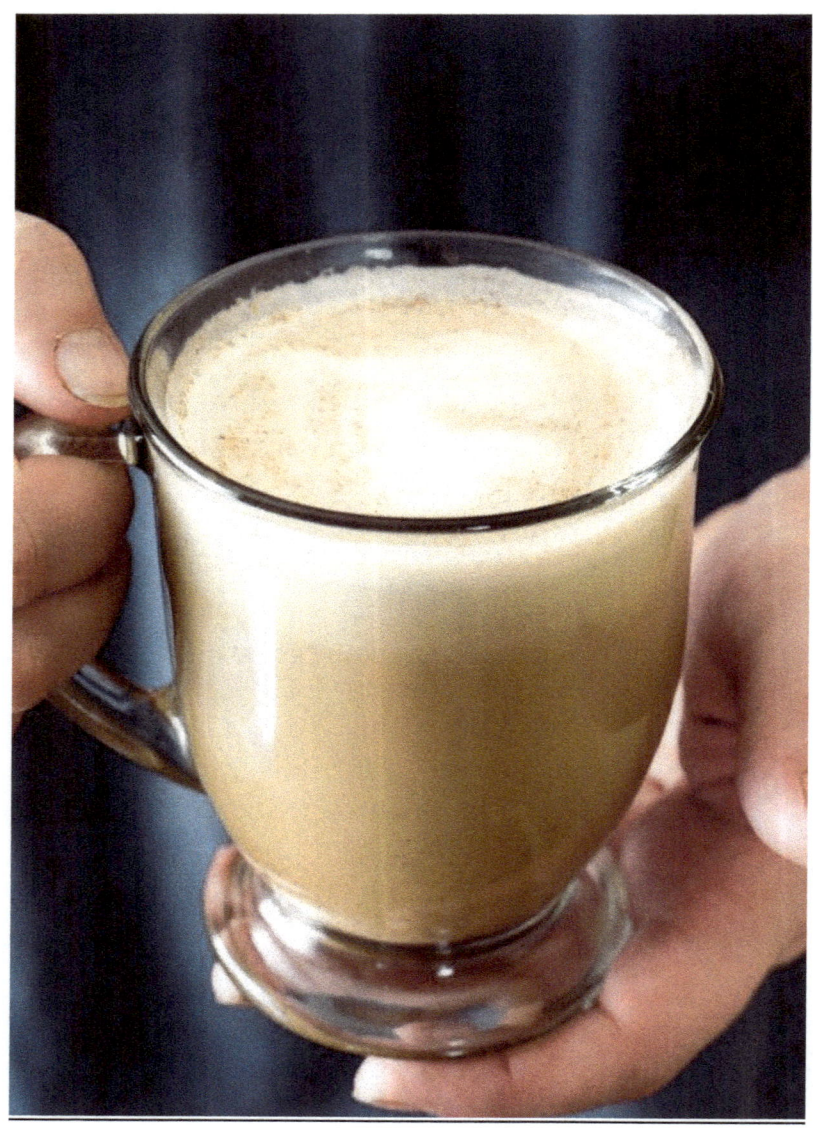

Preparation Time : 11 minutes

Cooking Time : 0 minute

Serving : 2

Ingredients :

- 2 cups almond milk
- ¼ cup coconut cream
- 2 teaspoons cannabis coconut oil
- ¼ cup pure pumpkin, canned
- ½ teaspoon vanilla extract
- 1 ½ teaspoon pumpkin spice
- ½ cup coconut whipped cream
- 1 pinch of salt

Directions :

1. Place all ingredients except the coconut whipped cream, in pan over a medium low heat stove.
2. Whisk well and allow to simmer but don't boil!
3. Simmer for about 5 minutes.
4. Pour into mugs and serve.

Nutrition : 94 Calories; 17g Carbohydrates; 3g Protein

Infused Turmeric-Ginger Tea

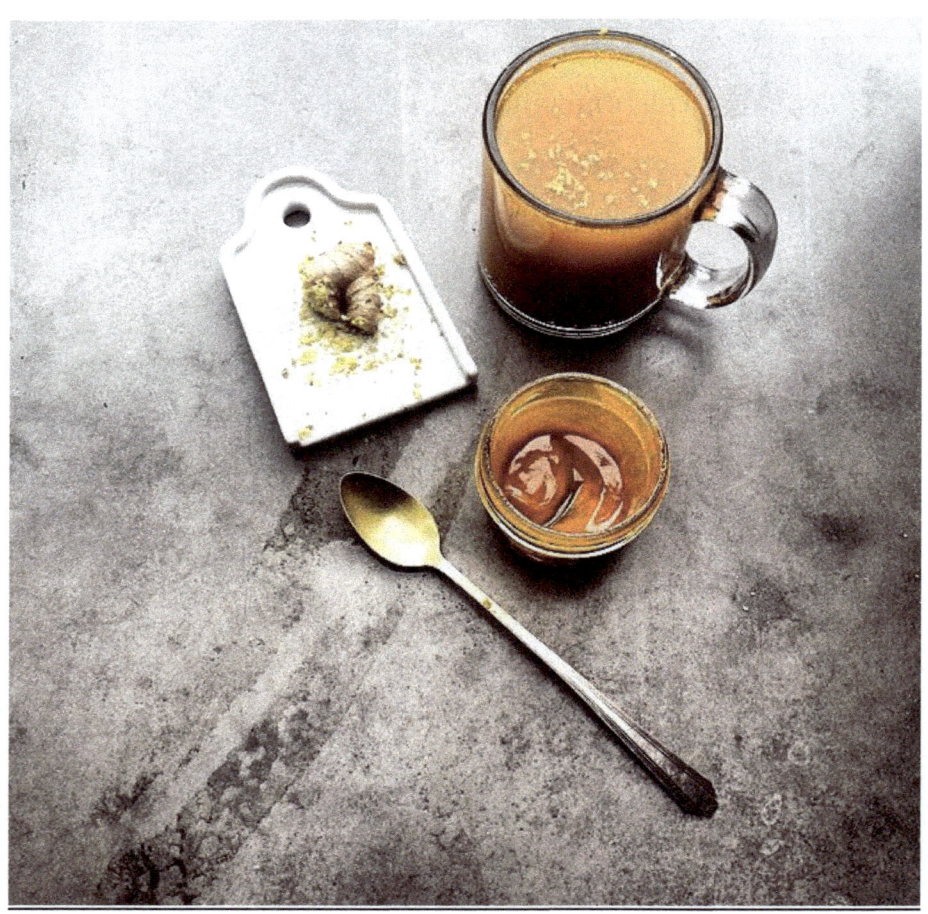

Preparation Time : 9 minutes

Cooking Time : 0 minute

Serving : 1

Ingredients :

- 1 cup water
- ½ cup coconut milk
- 1 teaspoon cannabis oil
- ½ teaspoon ground turmeric
- ¼ cup fresh ginger root, sliced
- 1 pinch Stevia or maple syrup, to taste

Directions :

1. Combine all ingredients in a small saucepan over medium heat.
2. Heat until simmer and turn heat low.
3. Take pan off the heat after 2 minutes
4. Let it cool, strain mixture into cup or mug.

Nutrition : 98 Calories; 14g Carbohydrates; 2g Protein

Infused London Fog

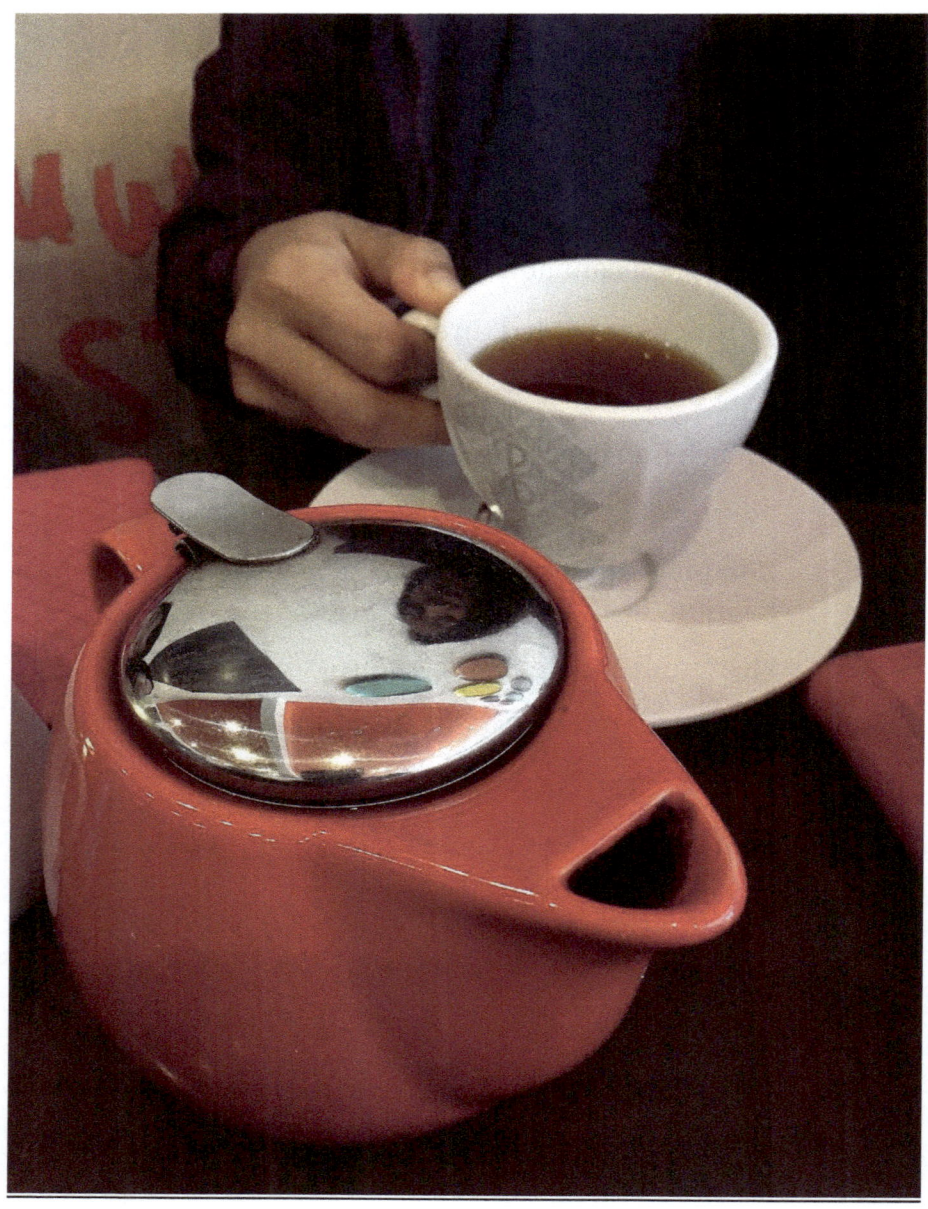

Preparation Time : 17 minutes

Cooking Time : 0 minute

Serving : 2

Ingredients :

- 1 cup hot water
- 1 Earl Grey teabag
- 1 teaspoon cannabis coconut oil
- ¼ cup almond milk
- ¼ teaspoon vanilla extract
- 1 pinch Stevia or sugar, to taste

Directions :

1. Fill up half a mug with boiling water.
2. Add teabag; if you prefer your tea strong, add two.
3. Add cannabis oil and stir well.
4. Add almond milk to fill your mug and stir through with the vanilla extract
5. Use Stevia or sugar to sweeten your Earl Grey to taste.

Nutrition : 76 Calories; 14g Carbohydrates; 2g Protein

Infused Cranberry-Apple Snug

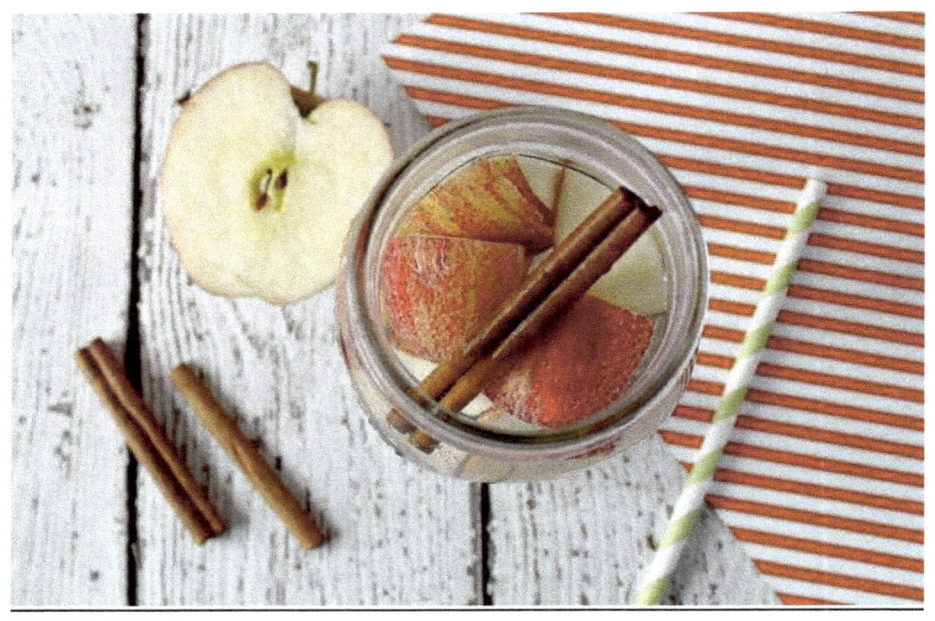

Preparation Time : 10 minutes

Cooking Time : 0 minute

Serving : 1

Ingredients :

- ½ cup fresh cranberry juice
- ½ cup fresh apple juice, cloudy
- ½ stick cinnamon
- 2 whole cloves
- ¼ lemon, sliced
- 1 pinch of Stevia or sugar, to taste
- cranberries for garnish (optional)

Directions :

1. Combine all ingredients in a small saucepan over medium heat.
2. Heat until simmer and turn heat low.
3. Let it cool, strain the mixture into a mug.
4. Serve with cinnamon stick and cranberries in a mug.

Nutrition : 88 Calories; 15g Carbohydrates; 3g Protein

Stomach Soother

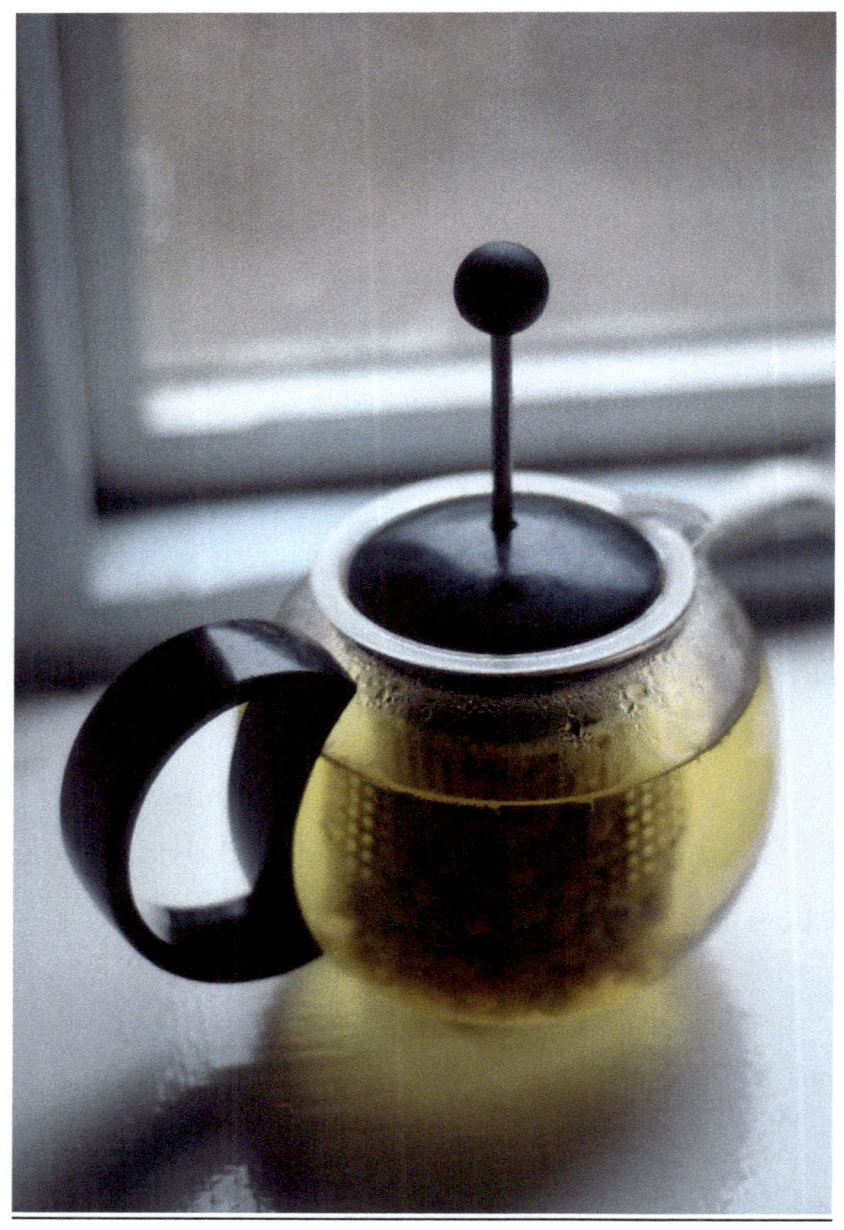

Preparation Time : 5 minutes

Cooking Time : 3 minutes

Servings : 1

Ingredients :

- Agave syrup, 1 tbsp.

- Ginger tea, .5 c

- Dr. Sebi's Stomach Relief Herbal Tea

- Burro banana, 1

Directions :

1. Fix the herbal tea according to the Directions on the package. Set it aside to cool.

2. Once the tea is cool, place it along with all the other Ingredients into a blender. Switch on the blender and let it run until it is creamy.

Nutrition :Calories 25; Sugar 3g; Protein 0.3g; Fat 0.5

Sarsaparilla Syrup

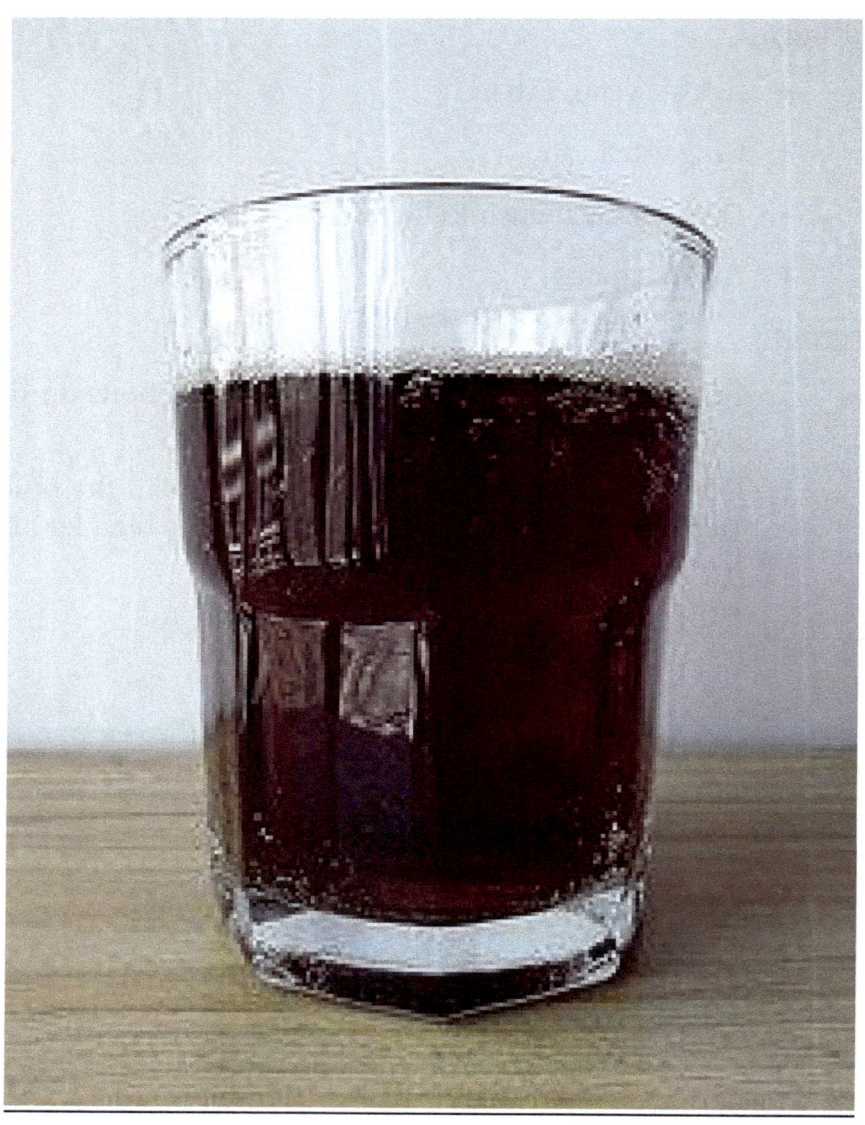

Preparation Time : 15 minutes

Cooking Time : 4 hours

Servings : 4

Ingredients :

- Date sugar, 1 c
- Sassafras root, 1 tbsp.
- Sarsaparilla root, 1 c
- Water, 2 c

Directions :

1. Firstly, add all of the Ingredients to a mason jar. Screw on the lid, tightly, and shake everything together. Heat a water bath up to 160. Sit the mason jar into the water bath and allow it to infuse for about two to four hours.

2. When the infusion time is almost up, set up an ice bath. Add half and half water and ice to a bowl. Carefully take the mason jar out of the water bath and place it into the ice bath. Allow it to sit in the ice bath for 15 to 20 minutes.

3. Strain the infusion out and into another clean jar.

Nutrition : Calories 37; Sugar 2g; Protein 0.4g; Fat 0.3

Dandelion "Coffee"

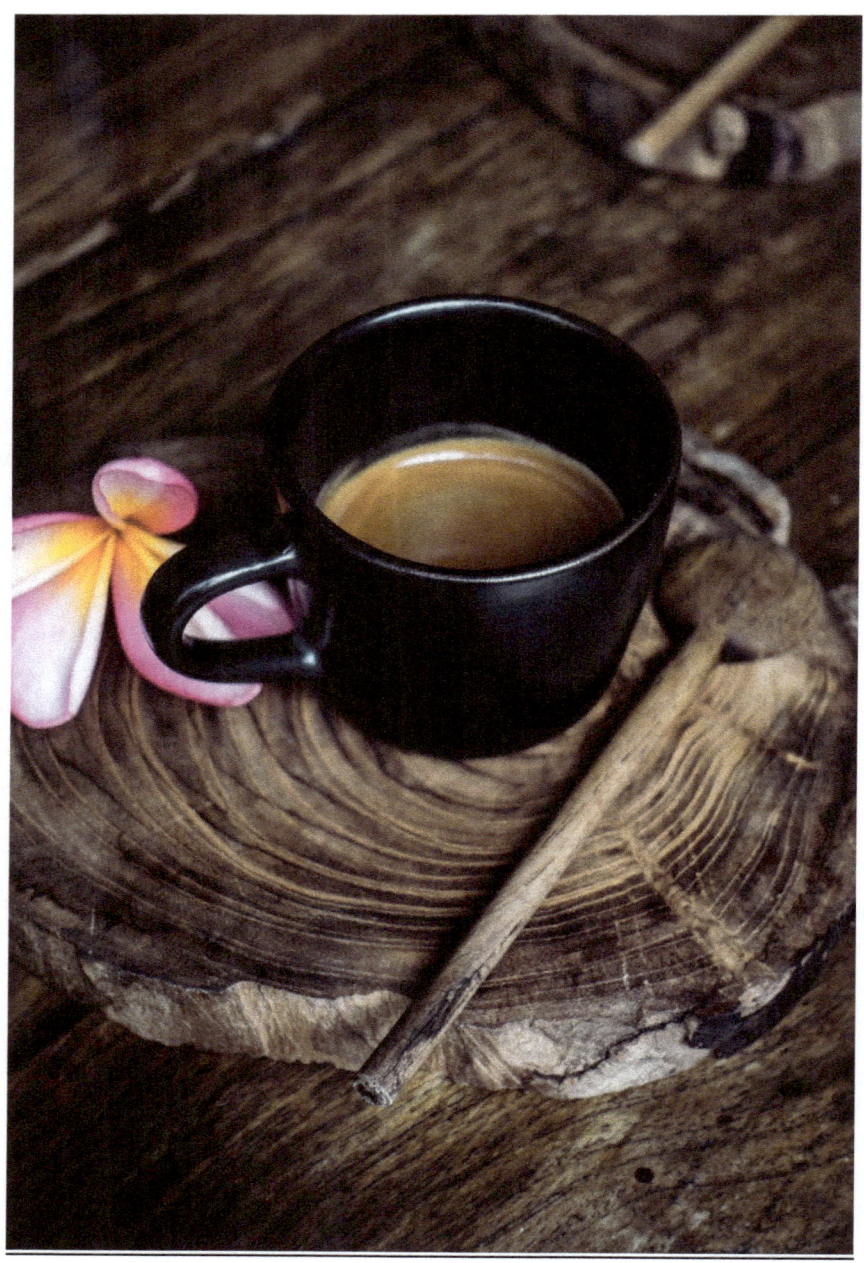

Preparation Time : 15 minutes

Cooking Time : 10 minutes

Servings : 4

Ingredients :

- Nettle leaf, a pinch

- Roasted dandelion root, 1 tbsp.

- Water, 24 oz.

Directions :

1. To start, we will roast the dandelion root to help bring out its flavors. Feel free to use raw dandelion root if you want to, but roasted root brings out an earthy and complex flavor, which is perfect for cool mornings.

2. Simply add the dandelion root to a pre-warmed cast iron skillet. Allow the pieces to roast on medium heat until they start to darken in color, and you start to smell their rich aroma. Make sure that you don't let them burn because this will ruin your teas taste.

3. As the root is roasting, have the water in a pot and allow it to come up to a full, rapid boil. Once your dandelion is roasted, add it to the boiling water with the nettle leaf. Steep this for ten minutes.

4. Strain. You can flavor your tea with some agave if you want to. Enjoy.

Nutrition : Calories 43; Sugar 1g; Protein 0.2g; Fat 0.3

Chamomile Delight

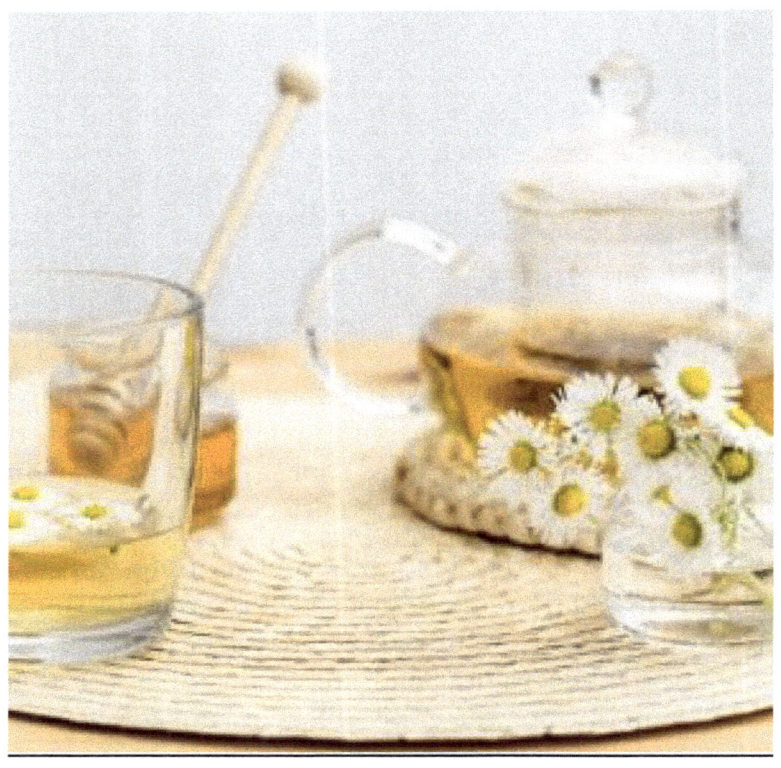

Preparation Time : 5 minutes

Cooking Time : 10 minutes

Servings : 3

Ingredients :

- Date sugar, 1 tbsp.
- Walnut milk, .5 c
- Dr. Sebi's Nerve/Stress Relief Herbal Tea, .25 c
- Burro banana, 1

Directions :

1. Prepare the tea according to the package Directions. Set to the side and allow to cool.

2. Once the tea is cooled, add it along with the above Ingredients to a blender and process until creamy and smooth.

Nutrition : Calories 21; Sugar 0.8g; Protein 1.0g; Fat 0.2g

Mucus Cleanse Tea

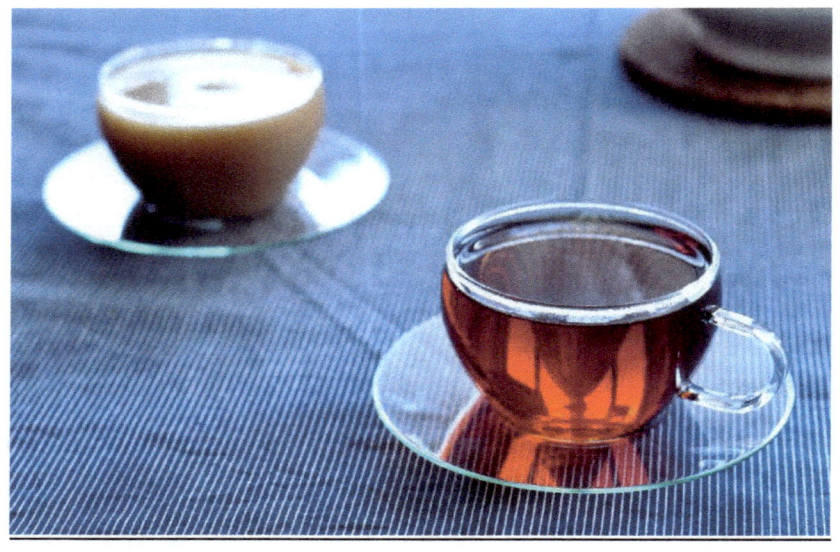

Preparation Time : 10 minutes

Cooking Time : 5 minutes

Servings : 2

Ingredients :

- Blue Vervain

- Bladder wrack

- Irish Sea Moss

Directions :

1. Add the sea moss to your blender. This would be best as a gel. Just make sure that it is totally dry.

2. Place equal parts of the bladder wrack to the blender. Again, this would be best as a gel. Just make sure that it is totally dry. To get the best results you need to chop these by hand.

3. Add equal parts of the blue vervain to the blender. You can use the roots to increase your iron intake and Nutritional healing values.

4. Process the herbs until they form a powder. This can take up to three minutes.

5. Place the powder into a non-metal pot and put it on the stove. Fill the pot half full of water. Make sure the herbs are totally immersed in water. Turn on the heat and let the liquid boil. Don't let it boil more than five minutes.

6. Carefully strain out the herbs. You can save these for later use in other recipes.

7. You can add in some agave nectar, date sugar, or key lime juice for added flavor.

Nutrition :Calories 36; Sugar 6g; Protein 0.7g; Fat 0.3g

Immune Tea

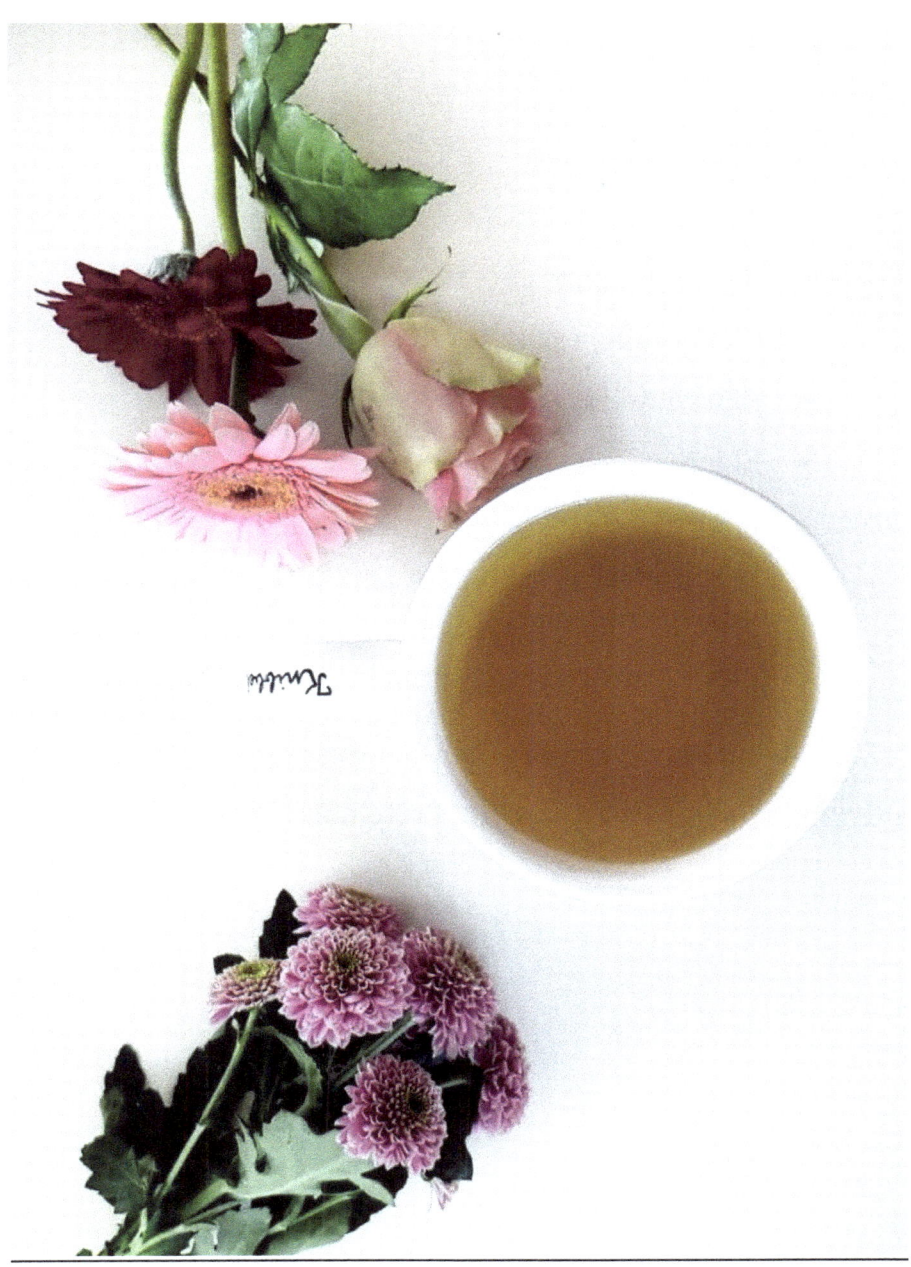

Preparation Time : 10 minutes

Cooking Time : 20 minutes

Servings : 1

Ingredients :

- Echinacea, 1 part
- Astragalus, 1 part
- Rosehip, 1 part
- Chamomile, 1 part
- Elderflowers, 1 part
- Elderberries, 1 part

Directions :

1. Mix the herbs together and place them inside an airtight container.

2. When you are ready to make a cup of tea, place one teaspoon into a tea ball or bag, and put it in eight ounces of boiling water. Let this sit for 20 minutes.

Nutrition : Calories 39; Sugar 1g; Protein 2g; Fat 0.6g

Ginger Turmeric Tea

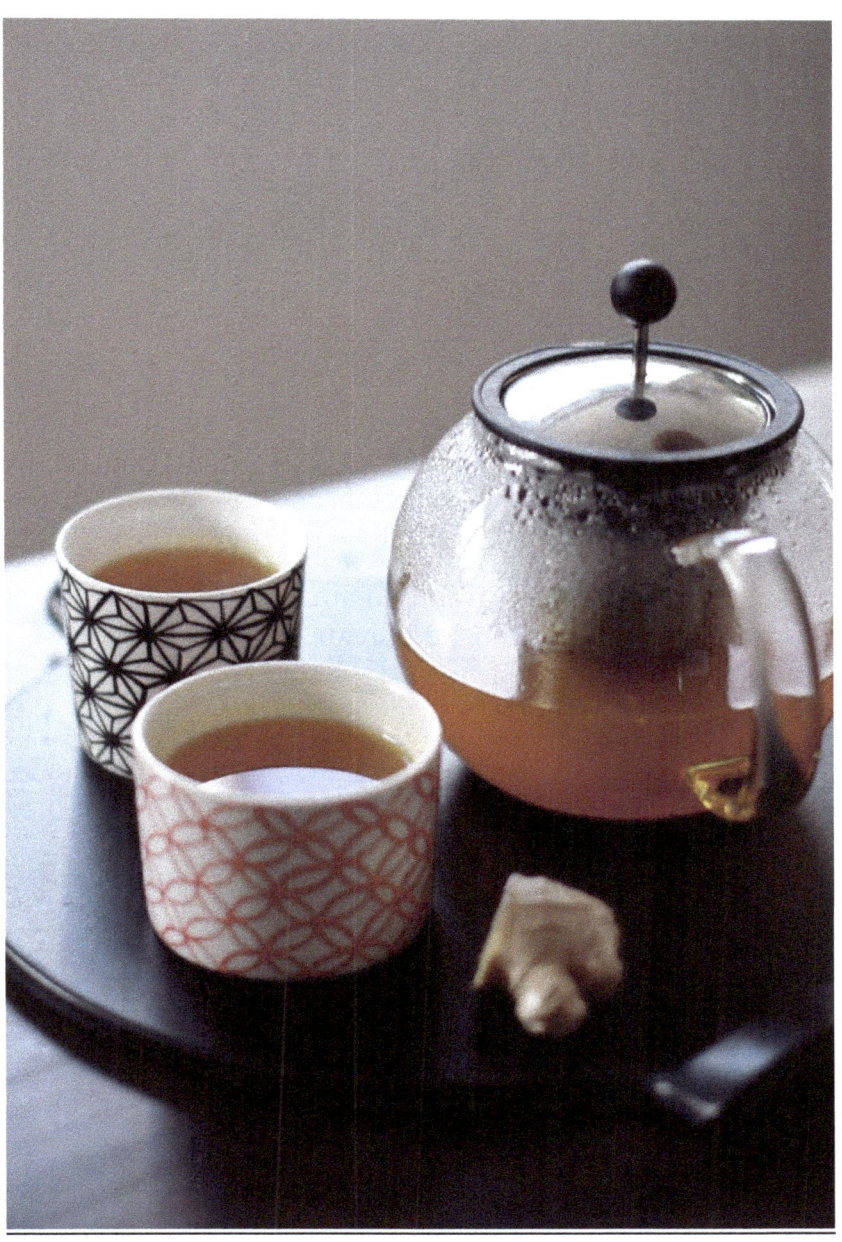

Preparation Time : 5 minutes

Cooking Time : 15 minutes

Servings : 2

Ingredients :

- Juice of one key lime
- Turmeric finger, couple of slices
- Ginger root, couple of slices
- Water, 3 c

Directions :

1. Pour the water into a pot and let it boil. Remove from heat and put the turmeric and ginger in. Stir well. Place lid on pot and let it sit 15 minutes.

2. While you are waiting on your tea to finish steeping, juice one key lime, and divide between two mugs.

3. Once the tea is ready, remove the turmeric and ginger and pour the tea into mugs and enjoy. If you want your tea a bit sweet, add some agave syrup or date sugar.

Nutrition : Calories 27; Sugar 5g; Protein 3g; Fat 1.0g

Tranquil Tea

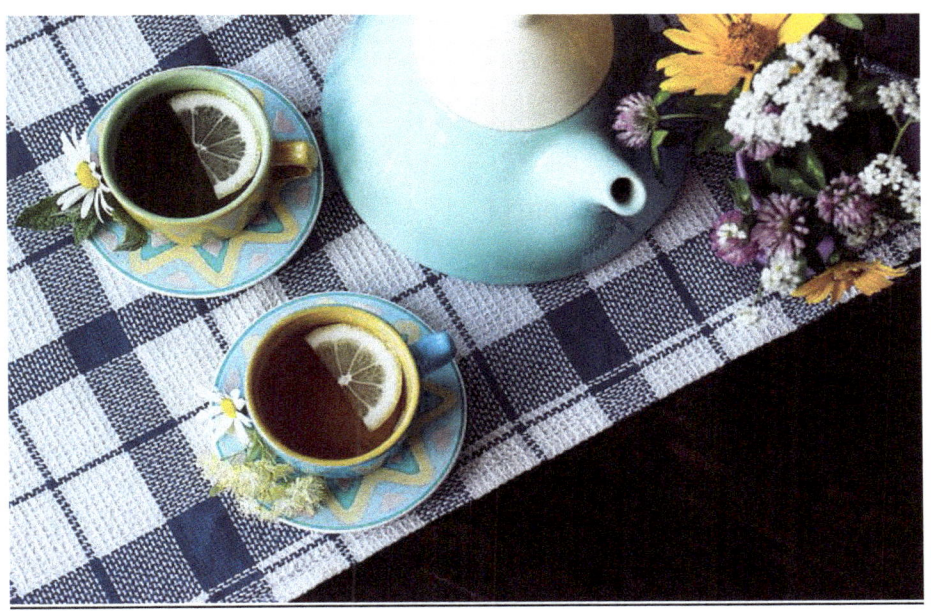

Preparation Time : 5 minutes

Cooking Time : 10 minutes

Servings : 2

Ingredients :

- Rose petals, 2 parts
- Lemongrass, 2 parts
- Chamomile, 4 parts

Directions :

1. Pour all the herbs into a glass jar and shake well to mix.

2. When you are ready to make a cup of tea, add one teaspoon of the mixture for every serving to a tea strainer, ball, or bag. Cover with water that has boiled and let it sit for ten minutes.

3. If you like a little sweetness in your tea, you can add some agave syrup or date sugar.

Nutrition :Calories 35; Sugar 3.4g; Protein 2.3g; Fat 1.5g

Energizing Lemon Tea

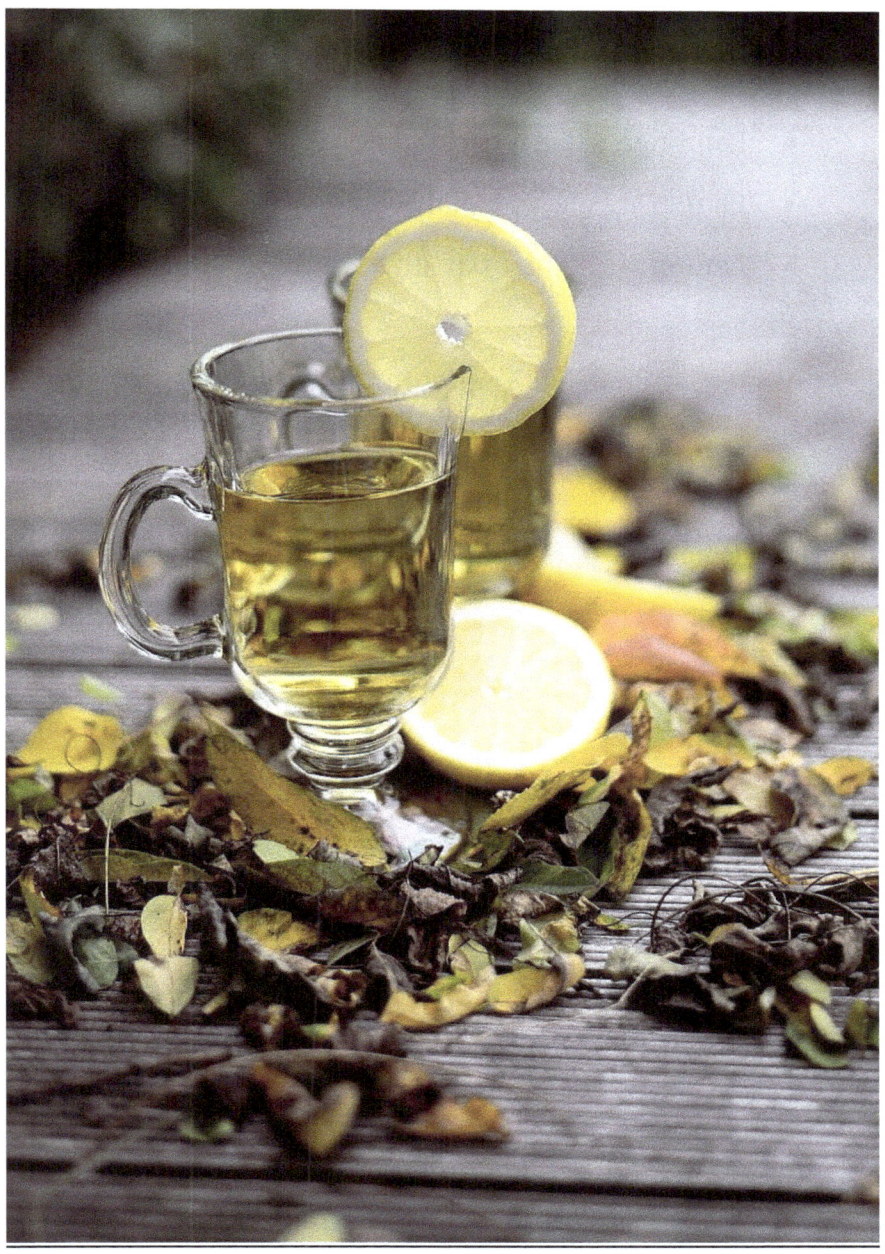

Preparation Time : 5 minutes

Cooking Time : 15 minutes

Servings : 3

Ingredients :

- Lemongrass, .5 tsp. dried herb
- Lemon thyme, .5 tsp. dried herb
- Lemon verbena, 1 tsp. dried herb

Directions :

1. Place the dried herbs into a tea strainer, bag, or ball and place it in one cup of water that has boiled. Let this sit 15 minutes. Carefully strain out the tea. You can add agave syrup or date sugar if needed.

Nutrition : Calories 40; Sugar 6g; Protein 2.2g; Fat 0.3